Trauma-Informed Yoga Therapy for Supporting
Asylum Seekers, Refugees, and New Immigrants

of related interest

Restorative Yoga for Ethnic and Race-Based Stress and Trauma
Gail Parker, Ph.D.
Illustrated by Justine Ross
Forewords by Octavia F. Raheem and Amy Wheeler, Ph.D.
ISBN 978 1 78775 185 9
eISBN 978 1 78775 186 6

Trauma Healing in the Yoga Zone
A Guide for Mental Health Professionals, Yoga Therapists and Teachers
Joann Lutz
Forewords by Arielle Schwartz and Sandra McLanahan
ISBN 978 1 91208 507 1
eISBN 978 1 91208 508 8

Trauma-Informed Yoga
Therapy for Supporting
ASYLUM SEEKERS, REFUGEES, AND NEW IMMIGRANTS

Gina M. Barrett with Mona Flynn

Foreword by Michael Lee

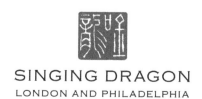

SINGING DRAGON
LONDON AND PHILADELPHIA

First published in Great Britain in 2025 by Singing Dragon,
an imprint of Jessica Kingsley Publishers
Part of John Murray Press

2

Four Lines by Rae Reed, LCS on page 25, reprinted with permission
from ArtLoveLifestyle magazine, Spring 2022

Photo credits: Whitley Marshall

Model credits: Patrick Kiruhura of Democratic Republic of the Congo, Marie
Manirakiza of Burundi, Whitley Marshall of Portland, Maine, USA

Front cover image source: Whitley Marshall. The cover image is for
illustrative purposes only, and any person featuring is a model.

A CIP catalogue record for this title is available from the
British Library and the Library of Congress

ISBN 978 1 80501 355 6
eISBN 978 1 80501 356 3

Printed and bound in Great Britain by CPI Group

Jessica Kingsley Publishers' policy is to use papers that are natural,
renewable and recyclable products and made from wood grown in
sustainable forests. The logging and manufacturing processes are expected
to conform to the environmental regulations of the country of origin.

Singing Dragon
Carmelite House
50 Victoria Embankment
London EC4Y 0DZ

www.singingdragon.com

John Murray Press
Part of Hodder & Stoughton Limited
An Hachette UK Company

The authorised representative in the EEA is Hachette Ireland,
8 Castlecourt Centre, Dublin 15, D15 XTP3, Ireland (email: info@hbgi.ie)

*To all the many donors, large and small, who
have made these programs possible.*

*To the gatekeepers who continue to welcome us to share
holistic trauma support with asylum seekers, refugees,
and new immigrants with trust and divine wisdom.*

Contents

Which type of seva is right for you?   115

Foreword

In my four decades of practicing and teaching yoga therapy, few developments have been as inspiring and transformative as the application of yoga to marginalized populations whose suffering often goes unaddressed by conventional therapies. Gina Barrett's work in *Trauma-Informed Yoga Therapy for Supporting Asylum Seekers, Refugees, and New Immigrants* stands as a testament to the power of yoga to heal profound wounds and restore dignity to those who have faced unimaginable challenges.

Gina's approach, rooted in the Phoenix Rising Method of Yoga Therapy, is a profound synthesis of ancient wisdom and modern therapeutic practice. I am honored that she chose this approach in this particular setting and am delighted to learn of the positive outcomes that resulted for so many of those with whom her team worked. The method facilitates deep embodied self-presence, guiding individuals towards inner peace, equanimity, and ease. It may initially seem paradoxical to encourage individuals who have endured deep trauma to reconnect with their bodies, yet the ancient yogis understood that the body holds a wisdom beyond the intellect—a truth that safety and well-being reside in the present moment, accessible through deep inner listening.

Gina and her team have applied these principles with refugees, asylum seekers, and immigrants, offering them profound experiences of healing and transformation. Their work exemplifies selfless service—yogic seva—in its purest form. Those offering it, as described in this book, do so from a place of profound presence and loving kindness. This, alone, is a catalyst for healing for those who have suffered.

Beyond the direct impact on individuals, Gina's contribution extends to offering a replicable model for others interested in engaging in this vital work. *Trauma-Informed Yoga Therapy for Supporting Asylum Seekers, Refugees, and New Immigrants* not only outlines a trauma-informed protocol but also provides essential guidance on establishing organizational structures to support these efforts sustainably. This includes practical insights into navigating the nonprofit sector, creating viable support systems, and mobilizing volunteers—all critical components in ensuring that yoga therapy reaches those most in need, regardless of their financial means.

This book is a comprehensive resource not only for yoga therapists and teachers but also for mental health professionals and medical practitioners seeking effective approaches to trauma healing in diverse cultural contexts. It addresses the complexities and challenges of offering yoga therapy to refugees, asylum seekers, and immigrants, making what may seem like a daunting endeavor appear feasible through detailed guidance and practical advice.

As we consider the profound impact of trauma on individuals and communities, the importance of trauma-informed care cannot be overstated. Gina's work offers a beacon of hope and practical wisdom, demonstrating that with dedication and the right framework, yoga therapy can be a transformative force for healing even in the most challenging circumstances.

This book dives into the world of nonprofit organizations and gives helpful, practical advice for those wishing to establish an appropriate organizational structure, purpose, and mission for the effective delivery of services to underserved communities, like refugees. There is a model here for those wishing to find one and adapt it to their unique needs.

In *Trauma-Informed Yoga Therapy for Supporting Asylum Seekers, Refugees, and New Immigrants* Gina M. Barrett invites us into a world where ancient wisdom meets contemporary compassion—a world where yoga becomes not just a physical practice but a path to reclaiming one's humanity and resilience. This book is not just a manual; it is a call to action for all those who believe in the healing potential of yoga and wish to make a meaningful difference in the lives of others.

May this book inspire and empower all who read it to embrace yoga as a tool for healing, compassion, and social change.

In loving service,

Michael Lee, MA, Dip.Soc.Sci., E-RYT, C-IAYT
Founder: Phoenix Rising Yoga Therapy

Introduction

Trauma-Informed Yoga Therapy, Yoga Therapy for
Trauma and the Global Immigration Crisis

Yoga therapy for mental health

Life brings us experiences that can radically change our behavior
as we seek to protect ourselves from harm. Phoenix Rising Yoga
Therapy (PRYT) is grounded in yoga and intersects with Buddhism,
psychology, and neuroscience. It seeks to support individuals in
restoring their own true nature and release fear. It does this through
a carefully facilitated process that takes them progressively from a
state of living in the mind to a state of deep embodied awareness in
the present moment—a safe place. This supports reconnection and
reintegration, first from an embodied felt sense, and then through
verbal facilitation to connect embodied experience to life experience.
It is a pro-symptom transformational approach to create a bridge
from body to soul. (Michael Lee, Founder of Phoenix Rising Yoga
Therapy, interviewed May 15, 2024)

As a practicing Phoenix Rising yoga therapist since 2003, I attract
clients who have experienced physical or sexual assault trauma, as
well as those with emotional trauma. All are choosing to transform
traumatic, lived experiences and overcome the effects they had on

their lives. With the support of a licensed mental health therapist, PRYT practitioners assist our clients in transforming trauma by facilitating awareness, acceptance, and new ways to respond when trauma may be reactivated.

Phoenix Rising yoga therapists use yoga, bodywork, witnessing, and dialog to help clients with mental health issues. Many of my clients come to me after doing talk therapy, realizing that their issues are more somatic. They notice the body–mind connection: that their emotions may be locked within their body and/or showing up as a physical or mental health ailment.

For example, someone with sexual assault trauma may experience numbness in their pelvis or unconsciously flinch when their partner approaches them with affection or sexual intentions. Some are so traumatized that they avoid being sexual. Others can respond by being overly sexual. This is what they were taught at a very young age, and the behavior becomes established in their brains.

Those physically abused as children may be choosing to transform their own tendencies to treat their children the way they were raised. Individuals with both physical and sexual abuse histories are also navigating post-traumatic stress disorder (PTSD). People who are physically abused may react to loud sounds and sudden movements. The same reactions can happen in those fleeing war zones.

In most cases, Phoenix Rising Yoga Therapy has catalyzed vast improvements in my clients. Body parts once numb awaken. Pain and chronic illness diminishes. Trauma reactions decrease and clients are able to function with more grace and ease in their daily lives.

As a witness and client-centered guide, holding one's client in a brave and safe container allows the client to safely open their physical body and *self-regulate* emotions and tensions that arise when talking about the abuse they experienced. *Self-regulation* is the use of self-care techniques or practices to bring oneself into a "window of tolerance" (see Chapter 2) where he/she/they can function less symptomatically. Be aware that follow-up with a mental health therapist may be required.

There is a process to all this, and it is best to go through the 1000-plus hour training to learn the techniques and practice your skills with professional feedback. Just a handful of schools offer yoga therapy for mental health. Each has its own unique approach to supporting those with mental health concerns.

Trauma-informed yoga therapy

There are many professional development trainings that offer shorter trauma-informed trainings for continued education. These are not the same as becoming a yoga therapist focused on mental health. These trauma-informed trainings are designed to help you instruct or practice as a yoga therapist with the awareness that your participants may have experienced trauma in one form or another to varying degrees. With this awareness, you can share self-regulation techniques and tools that will support your participants in self-regulating their trauma symptoms.

By its nature, yoga can activate emotions and trauma symptoms. We are stretching muscle and connective tissue that may have been held as a trauma response for years, even decades. Holding, contracting, or numbing body parts, and blocking traumatic memories in the mind, is how the body and mind protect themselves. These are primitive and involuntary brain responses to survival issues, explained in more detail later in this book. When these body parts are released in a brave, safe, and supportive setting, emotions and memories can surface. It is important to know what not to do when this happens while teaching or when providing a yoga therapy consult.

Immigration and mental health

According to recent statistics, mental illness is on the rise in the US and worldwide. In the United States, the Centers for Disease Control and Prevention's National Center for Injury Prevention and Control (2024) states that...

Mental illnesses are among the most common health conditions in the United States.

- More than 1 in 5 US adults live with a mental illness.

- Over 1 in 5 youth (ages 13–18) either currently or at some point during their life, have had a seriously debilitating mental illness.

- About 1 in 25 US adults lives with a serious mental illness, such as schizophrenia, bipolar disorder, or major depression.

There is no single cause for mental illness. A number of factors can contribute to risk for mental illness, such as

- Adverse childhood experiences, such as trauma or a history of abuse (for example, child abuse, sexual assault, witnessing violence, etc.)

- Experiences related to other ongoing (chronic) medical conditions, such as a traumatic brain injury, cancer, or diabetes

- Biological factors or chemical imbalances in the brain

- Use of alcohol or drugs

- Having feelings of loneliness or isolation

And according to the World Health Organization...

In 2019 970 million people globally were living with a mental disorder, with anxiety and depression the most common.

Mental health conditions can cause difficulties in all aspects of life, including relationships with family, friends, and community. They can result from or lead to problems at school and at work.

Globally, mental disorders account for 1 in 6 years lived with disability. People with severe mental health conditions die 10 to

20 years earlier than the general population. And having a mental health condition increases the risk of suicide and experiencing human rights violations.

The economic consequences of mental health conditions are also enormous, with productivity losses significantly outstripping the direct costs of care. (World Health Organization, n.d.)

The Refugee Health Technical Assistance Center (2024) has found that the more common mental health diagnoses associated with refugee populations include PTSD, major depression, generalized anxiety, panic attacks, adjustment disorder, and somatization. Rates of PTSD and major depression in settled adult refugees range from 10% to 40% and 5% to 15%, respectively, while children and adolescents have rates of PTSD as high as 50% to 90% and major depression ranging from 6% to 40%. Refugees may also suffer from panic attacks, adjustment disorder, and somatization. According to the Center, the number of traumas someone has experienced, [along with] delayed asylum application process, detention, and the loss of culture and support systems all contribute to the risk of developing mental health problems.

During six years running a nonprofit, Casa de Paz San Luis Valley (SLV), whose mission is to provide holistic trauma support for asylum seekers, refugees, and new immigrants internationally, I have seen that our participants often experienced many of the causes for mental illness listed above, especially "trauma history from abuse," poverty, displacement, and "feelings of loneliness and isolation." Examples include loss of family members due to war, natural disasters or gang violence, family separation, human trafficking, kidnapping, sexual and physical assault, and declining health and high stress due to poverty.

When someone experiences multiple traumas in their lifetime, their mental health condition is considered "complex trauma." Individuals who have experienced many traumatic events in their lifetime can have many different responses when trauma is reactivated by day-to-day life experiences, like loud sounds, unexpected contact, or movements around them, or other experiences that reactivate past traumatic experiences, memories, and more.

Notice that I intentionally choose not to use the word "trigger" because of its violent root. I use the word "activate" instead.

In this book, we will go into more detail about evidence-based complex trauma responses, how they occur in the body, and how yoga therapy can assist in co-regulation and self-regulation. *Co-regulation* happens when the clients is learning self-regulation techniques with a teacher or other students. The nervous system regulates with the assistance of, or in the presence of, the teacher or group. All present experience the benefits of the practice.

Most people do not make mental health a priority. In some cultures, mental health challenges are considered an embarrassment, failure, or weakness, and is handled only within the family. I have found this to be the case in the Latinx culture that we primarily serve at Casa de Paz SLV. Getting mental health support is often seen as a privilege and also handled within the family. As we serve as yoga instructors and yoga therapists in these marginalized communities, we need to be aware of this. Often people's lives are so difficult, as they struggle to survive, that they are unable to find time or energy to attend a free support group, even if they know they need it and want to heal. The same goes for accessing any resources that may be available. A little assistance can go a long way in the lives of these individuals. Seva, or selfless service, and multicultural sensitivity are also major considerations and are discussed in more detail in Chapter 2.

The stress of poverty, living with trauma symptoms, and displacement are the lived experience of most new immigrants, refugees in encampments, and migrants. They are exhausted and struggling to survive with very little money or support. It is very difficult to survive in the United States on the US minimum wage or even $20 per hour. Many new immigrants pile into family or friend's homes with no privacy, several people to a room, everyone shares one computer, etc. Most have exhausting labor-intensive jobs and children at home that require care. The stresses of poverty, such as low-quality food and access to quality healthcare are very real for them.

So, how do these individuals access mental healthcare? This is what we have been doing at the border of Texas and Mexico since 2019. We have also done some online trauma support and training in the Dzaleka Refugee Camp in Malawi, Africa, which houses over 50,000 refugees struggling to survive with limited resources and surrounded by corruption. While migrants wait to cross over into the US or for sponsorship to resettle, we can help them learn self-regulation skills to assist them with trauma symptoms from their immigration journey or refugee experience.

Prior to 2019, as a Phoenix Rising yoga therapist, I had primarily served those who could pay out-of-pocket or offer professional trades. With a Master's degree in International Administration and my experience working in developing countries, when the border crisis started showing up in the news, I could not help but notice the trauma that asylum seekers experienced on their immigration journey. What was shared in the news was that asylum seekers often endure sexual and physical assault, natural disaster, and war-zone trauma. It soon became clear to me that there was a mass movement of traumatized people coming into the United States. These people would need help with self-regulation in order to function in their daily lives. It was time to be of service to those who have nothing.

In 2022, the International Organization for Migration reported that:

> [t]he number of global migrants is increasing slightly faster than the world's population: They represent 3.3 percent of all people today, compared with 2.6 percent in 1960, according to United Nations statistics. Overall, the estimated number of international migrants has increased over the past five decades. The total estimated 281 million people living in a country other than their countries of birth in 2020 was 128 million more than in 1990 and over three times the estimated number in 1970. (2022)

We are now seeing an increase in immigration into the United States and Europe. This is the result of gang violence, political unrest, economic inequities, and climate change affecting food sources and housing. Over the past five years, the US is seeing larger numbers of asylum seekers and refugees from Central America, the Gaza Strip, Afghanistan, Ukraine, Mexico, the Dzaleka Refugee Camp in Malawi, Africa, Syria, Haiti, Israel, Venezuela, and other countries in Asia and Africa. Because of the wide range of languages spoken, nonverbal communication skills for sharing trauma-informed yoga are needed.

In the following chapters, contributor Mona Flynn and I will share how yoga therapy can help to self-regulate trauma symptoms. We will also share the programs we have created for asylum seekers, refugees, and new immigrants. Not only do we provide evidence-based trauma-informed yoga therapy sequences, but we also share how to create a trauma-informed yoga program, along with suggestions for creating a nonprofit. May all this information be of service. We are also available as trainers and consultants to guide you deeper into this service when you are ready.

The lives of migrants and refugees

Casa de Paz SLV worked in partnership with the MUTU (Me You Together for Union) organization in the Dzaleka Refugee Camp in Malawi, Africa. In the encampment, these refugees have little hope of immigrating to a new country, unless they can find a sponsor who can pay their way. Corruption exists around this process as well; for example, being told that paying a bribe is necessary, not knowing if the person offering the passports and entry into a new country will follow through. The risks include kidnapping or even enslavement. In the meantime, corruption also exists regarding distribution of rations. For this reason, and because of drought, hunger, and starvation, suicide rates are very high. There are also limited medical supplies for the very painful sickle cell anemia that is endemic there.

GUNSHOTS

In the head of this mom
"No! Take everything, but leave me alive."
"Please take everything, but leave me alive,"
she screamed but none to hear.
None to say, "sorry." Those died...none could bury
Listen "PA!PA!PA!PA!"
This is how it goes to be a refugee. I am a refugee.
Yes, I am a refugee. I didn't choose to be.
I have reasons that made me flee. Real
Tell me your story
Such a question does not fit me
I'm no longer me
Citizenship and passport no longer exist in me

My status has made everyone my enemy
Asylum seeker my economy
Handout my Salary

Day after day I'm taught of sanctuary
Tell no one my ration
Refugees are broken nations
Tears, gunshots and vomit that's me

A refugee is just a human being like you in a foreign country

Out of fear of political persecution, natural disasters, and many more.
Take care of them and don't treat them as animal

Let's not hear of this anymore

NTABE MUGALIHYA, AGE 22, CONGOLESE REFUGEE AT
DZALEKA REFUGEE CAMP IN MALAWI, AFRICA, 2015–24

Since I began serving at the border of Texas and Mexico in 2019–21, the numbers of asylum seekers went from approximately a hundred waiting for entry into the United States at the Brownsville & Matamoros International Bridge, to upwards of three thousand migrants. An encampment was built there with the input of the migrants, mostly from countries in Central America, as well as Cuba. The large encampment was proudly maintained by migrants and many volunteer organizations. The city of Matamoros and the Mexican government were supportive for a while, but the encampment was soon dismantled. Some migrants went to shelters. Others were determined to cross into the United States after their long journey to the border and caravanned to the closest point of entry, Reynosa, Mexico.

Thousands piled up in tent cities in this remote and dangerous location during the COVID-19 pandemic. It was very difficult for the relief organizations supporting the migrants in Matamoros to help in Reynosa, but some continued as best as they could. Read the article below, written by our board chair (2021–4), Rae Reed, LCSW in Chicago, who traveled to Reynosa with Sister Norma of Catholic Charities, and again with Casa de Paz SLV, leading a team of trauma support volunteers.

Now, migrants continue to arrive in Matamoros, Mexico, where a small, very unsanitary encampment was built. Most of the migrants are bused inland to shelters. On my last service trip, in January 2024, some (approximately 150 adults and children) chose to take the risk of unsanitary and unsafe conditions here, to be closer to services, work opportunities, and the bridge into the United States. They prefer to be able to move freely and independently on foot. One thing that is guaranteed is that the temporary infrastructure is always changing at the border. What is set up for migrants now may be very different from what will be set up a few months from now. Flexibility is a necessary skill to cultivate while working in this environment.

FOUR LINES

by Rae Reed, LCSW

Lines...a reality that migrants at the U.S./Mexico border know all too well—lines for food, lines for clothes, lines for a shower. In autumn of 2022, on my trip to the border with Casa De Paz SLV, I witnessed how the fates of asylum seekers were determined by the line they were allowed to wait in.

When working with unaccompanied minors in Brownsville, Texas, I witnessed the line of order. One that the children were accustomed to: the "fila" to get to a field trip, a meal, school or recreation outside. This line was temporary, a way to quickly count heads and enforce rules. With increased numbers of unaccompanied minors crossing over the border, the enforcement of these lines becomes paramount. Staff members felt the weight of their role knowing they were responsible for keeping each one of these kids safe, a lot of whom were being reunited with their families.

In an unaccompanied minor's shelter, just like in detention for adults, a line can serve as a reminder of captivity, even if that captivity is temporary. That captivity was felt but superseded by the ties each child had, to each other and their families. Some talked of their own children as being motivating factors. Others discussed music as being a guiding force through this time. One was an avid drummer. Their taste in music varied from Creedence Clearwater to Bad Bunny. Their artwork in which they were asked to reflect on their identity and their identity in relation to others mirrored this variety.

In Reynosa, Mexico, where we served for the majority of our final day, a line meant three things. In the plaza where thousands waited for legal consultation, a line meant desperation. As we passed a line of over one hundred people standing in the bright sun adjacent to the weather-worn tents they lived in, one man asked us for legal consult. Those in line were seeking the same.

The dirt on children's clothing, the lack of food and sanitary items and the absence of organized humanitarian support communicated that the conditions in this location were far worse than those that had previously existed in Matamoros, Mexico. An extra variable asylum seekers contended with in Reynosa was fear of robbery, rape, assault, and kidnapping. Desperation was an understatement as families crowded around our bus pressing the pastor who ran the shelter to give them a way out of that situation. A seven-year-old boy and his mother had been kidnapped while living in the plaza in Reynosa and were now in the shelter awaiting their asylum claim.

Outside the shelter in Reynosa, a line meant exasperation. Upon our arrival, we witnessed large crowds of hundreds of migrants from Central America, South America, and Haiti waiting outside for their chance to stay in this shelter. They were surrounded by run-down shacks that they were paying rent to live in, as their name progressed down the long waiting list that was their only ticket into this location.

The coveted aspect of this shelter: a gate that separated them from the danger that Reynosa posed. Though most of the migrants in the shelter remained outside in tents, they were provided some amenities that those in the plaza didn't have, such as three meals a day and bathrooms that included showers.

While doing relational-based artwork with children and their parents, a few asylum seekers in the shelter were rifling through the belongings that were left behind. Some were seeking a clean T-shirt or pair of underwear. This communicated that even when in a desired location, asylum seekers still lacked basic necessities.

The children with whom we did art therapy often presented as older than their age as the compounded obstacles of the journey, the persecution they experienced at home, and the challenges of living outside in Mexico caused them to grow up too soon. When they were asked if they were leaving that day, they would say "Mañana, si Dios permite," (Tomorrow if God allows it). It was clearly a phrase their parents used to temper their child's expectations in a situation where anything could change moment by moment. But coming out of an eight-year-old's mouth, it communicated a maturity that was earned but not desired. Because of this, the chance to be kids for a moment was inviting, whether that meant drawing pictures for their "Art teacher" or pretending their yoga mat was a race car.

It was clear each child was looking for connection. As a therapist, I have learned just how much relationships can be a stabilizing force in the wake of trauma. Drawing and yoga were a conduit for those relationships, in which drawing a flower, or a house could lead to a deeper conversation about how to have a sense of belonging in a place where they were given the message that they don't belong. The impact of these relationships was shown in the amount of time each child spent completing art and their readiness to try yoga, an activity not commonly practiced by most of the families we served. After trauma-informed yoga, one Haitian boy was found practicing the tree pose on his own next to his tent. I could see how he connected to it, a small part of his world that he could control when his asylum status was something he could not.

Adults looking for calm and serenity benefited from yoga and massage therapy. One man encouraged another to join yoga, saying that it helped relax his mind from the worries he felt so frequently in the shelter. Many complained of ailments, like chronic headaches, diabetes and muscle tension. We offered massage therapy, medicinal teas and essential oils as natural remedies that could aid any medical support they were already getting. Doctors without Borders had visited this shelter, and through the questions asylum seekers asked, it was clear they thought we were healthcare professionals and were looking for further medical care. In the process of informing them we weren't, we learned that one woman was diabetic without access to any insulin.

In the backdrop of all these experiences was the final kind of line: the line of hope. When we first arrived at the shelter, there was a line of families with backpacks and suitcases in front of a school bus that would take them across the border legally. We gave families snacks and water bottles for their journey. In the five-hour period that we were in Reynosa, three busloads of families were brought over to the United States.

Towards the end of the day, I was waiting in the church's outdoor courtyard when a line of fifty people walked to the bus that would take them out of the holding pattern in Reynosa into a line where they were walking forward toward their end goal in McAllen, Texas. Those who had to remain cheered and clapped, letting go of their anguish for a moment to celebrate with their friends. Elation was the feeling I sensed from them as they hurried quickly to collect their belongings. The atmosphere was jubilant, creating a levity that was scarce in this border town, one they wished to be the rule rather than the exception.

Of all the lines I experienced that weekend, this one was by far the best. The type of line asylum seekers came all this way to get in. It didn't exempt them from being in other lines, like the line to asylum status for example, but it kept them from gambling with their life in a line that they did not choose. That simple act of agency, something those who experienced trauma gravely need, can so often be the necessary link in the progression between despair and hope in the life of a new immigrant.

Our service continues as holistic trauma-informed retreats in Crestone, Colorado, as well as online support for asylum seekers and new immigrants.

Rae Reed, LCSW (he/him) from Chicago and Casa de Paz SLV Board Chair (2021–4) has been working with refugees and asylum seekers for many years in private agencies. Rae has led many service trips to the border encampments. Rae's hope is that one day soon asylum seekers will be able to safely await their asylum cases in the United States.

Reprinted with permission from ArtLoveLifestyle
magazine, Spring 2022

What is seva?

According to yoga philosophy, seva, selfless service, is an integral part of the yoga lifestyle. When we serve, we burn karma that has been accumulated over lifetimes. I can attest to this, because, once I started doing this work in a serious and completely selfless way, I was provided for in many ways. I was given speaking opportunities, discounts, trainings, and lodging. Volunteers were attracted to us to help. Yoga studio owners put donation cans in their studios and sent donation checks with what they collected from their students. We had donation patrons who sent checks monthly. Doors opened for Casa de Paz SLV easily to serve at the border of Texas and Mexico and in the Dzaleka Refugee Camp in Malawi Africa. I felt a clearing in my interpersonal relationships. People who had once wronged me in the past were donating large sums of money and/

or sending volunteers. I don't take this for granted and made sure I continued to operate the nonprofit with a high level of integrity, always keeping the yoga sutras in mind. Seva is a priority in organizations such as Yoga Alliance and the International Association of Yoga Therapists, and funding and recognition are provided for seva projects.

CHAPTER 1

Theory and Practice: Applying Trauma-Informed Yoga to Asylum Seeker, Refugee, and Immigrant Populations

Contribution by Mona Hibawi Flynn, Doctoral Candidate, EdD, C-IAYT

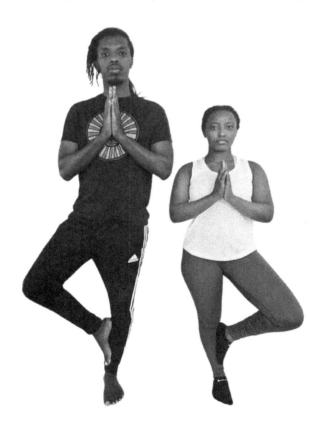

Trauma and immigrant/refugee populations

Since the US Congress passed the 1980 Refugee Act, nearly three million refugees have resettled in the United States (Kumar, Soffer, & Begg 2021). Refugees are defined as those who are unable to return to their home countries due to a well-founded fear of persecution due to race, religion, nationality, membership in a particular social group, or political opinion (Global Migration Data Analysis Centre 2024). Most often they have been forced to flee their homeland abruptly, unable to return home due to safety issues. Upon obtaining refugee status from organizations like the United Nations, international laws provide protection and life-saving support through different agencies (US Department of State: Bureau of Population, Refugees, and Migration n.d.). Refugees in the United States can legally become permanent residents and eventually citizens through established protocol. Asylum seekers, though seeking international protection from dangers and their homeland, have not yet legally obtained refugee status. They apply for protection with the country of their destination once they arrive at or cross the border. In the United States, meeting criteria for refugee protection involves following US and international laws, and includes going before a court to explain one's case. It is usually very stressful, since timetables vary and are costly for individual(s) who do not yet have a home or employment. Immigrants are individuals who have decided to leave their home country and move to another country with the intention of settling. Often they become lawful permanent residents, seeking employment and other opportunities. They must also go through a vetting process, free to return to their home country whenever they choose.

The healthcare demographics of immigrants, refugees, and asylum seekers are affected by migration patterns in response to worldwide conflicts and health-related developments. A study by the United Nations Refugee Agency's Annual Global Trends Analysis revealed that, by the end of 2016, 65.6 million individuals had experienced involuntary displacement across the globe (Müller *et al.* 2018). The evolving global COVID–19 pandemic, disruptive changes in governments, and war have contributed to unexpected migration patterns since early 2020. Trajectories of the many different groups of migrants and refugees evolved from survival efforts and involve health-related factors including nutrition, shelter, clean water, and safety. The interplay of such factors specific to each group and individual, significantly shapes the health profiles of asylum seekers, often diverging from those of their home country, due to experiences prior to emigration, refugee camps, transit to the host nation, and residence in asylum centers, predisposing them to psychological issues and increased susceptibility to infectious diseases (Müller *et al.* 2018). These endured traumas precipitate myriad physical, emotional, and mental challenges, complicating medical treatment on multiple fronts, including language barriers, intercultural communication hurdles, and the integration of asylum seekers into the healthcare system (Müller *et al.* 2018).

Forced or involuntary migration includes both conflict-induced and disaster-induced displacement. The definitions of these concepts are used in the documentation of an individual's history, which then determines qualification for various aid resources, recognizing unique circumstances essential to meeting immediate needs, as well as for long range successful resettlement to ensure improving quality of life. Vital to successful resettlement are welcoming communities where organizations and caring individuals are willing to help bridge the gaps to enable access to existing resources, as well as to provide unmet essential needs.

Immigrant populations often initially exhibit better health upon arrival in the United States compared to the general populace. However, with prolonged residence, they tend to adopt cardiovascular risk profiles resembling those of the native population. This decline, especially noticeable among women, is attributed in part to decreased physical activity and poorer dietary habits post-immigration (Wieland *et al.* 2012). Epidemiological data underscore the prevalence of chronic diseases and physical inactivity among culturally and linguistically diverse (CALD) migrants as they navigate cultural and modernization shifts (Caperchione, Kolt, & Mummery 2009). Despite greater susceptibility to chronic illnesses, individuals from CALD backgrounds may not always seek healthcare or engage in preventive measures for optimal health outcomes (Wegnelius & Petersson 2018; Westgard *et al.* 2021).

Barriers to preventive self-care faced by CALD groups

Migration to Western societies can adversely impact the health, and health-sustaining behaviors of CALD groups as they adjust to new environments, cultures, and lifestyles. Various challenges, such as cultural beliefs, social issues, economic disparities, environmental factors, and perceptions of health and injury hinder their access to physical and mental healthcare (Caperchione *et al.* 2009). Trauma can further disconnect individuals from their bodies, affecting their ability to perceive physical sensations and attend to health needs. Overcoming these barriers requires culturally sensitive approaches, education on health behaviors, community support, affordable preventive healthcare options, and targeted health programs. Addressing these issues is crucial for improving the physical and mental well-being of CALD populations (Caperchione *et al.* 2009).

Government aid for meeting the needs of resettling includes social services, assessing immediate health needs, and providing access to language learning, education, and essential needs; yet, most of these services are temporary, relying on local communities to continue to support newcomers and on the migrants themselves to acclimatize and become independent. Despite emerging support systems, not all migrant groups understand what is available. Some are undocumented citizens who do not have access to services, and whose barriers to care are well beyond those who are documented. In all these ways, immigrants miss opportunities for learning about options to help themselves and their families. As the focus on daily survival continues, self-care is not recognized as a priority.

Potential benefits of yoga therapy for immigrants/refugees living with PTSD

Immigrants and refugees may have ongoing mental health concerns, such as PTSD and depression, due to repeated and varying trauma experienced before, during, and after fleeing their country of origin (Kumar *et al.* 2021). Although healthcare provisions and community-based mental health interventions aim to improve physical and mental health outcomes among immigrants and refugees in the United States, these services are underutilized (Kumar *et al.* 2021).

Movement-based and mind-body-focused practices, such as yoga and yoga therapy, may play an important role as complementary mental health support (Sengupta 2012). Traumas of the past are replaced with the healing that happens from physical strengthening as well as from the psychosocial health improvements from newly cultivated relationships. In this manner, yoga is being introduced as a simple and economical therapeutic modality that may be considered a beneficial adjuvant to psychotherapy (Mitchell *et al.* 2014; Nickerson *et al.* 2011). Data on the effectiveness of these interventions in these populations are limited, and further research is needed. However, these practices can still be introduced in a safe way by trained professionals and offered as therapeutic approaches to traditional Western psychotherapy options (Kumar *et al.* 2021).

Theoretical models for trauma-informed yoga

The vast interdisciplinary umbrella of neuroscience research looks to document the effects of mind-body practices from the physical to the subtle layers of the body, to be understood even at cellular levels. Scientific research applies theoretical models to explore and edify traditionally preventative uses of mind-body modalities. The following current models offer interwoven explanations of mind-body modalities for resilience and post-traumatic growth:

- the modern scientific model of polyvagal theory

- the ancient panchamaya kosha model from yoga philosophy

- the ancient gunas model from Ayurveda.

Polyvagal theory

Polyvagal theory identifies three branches of the autonomic nervous system (ANS): the ventral vagal, sympathetic, and dorsal vagal systems. Understanding how these systems function and interact is crucial in tailoring trauma-sensitive mind-body practices (Porges 2022). Trauma dysregulates three parts of the ANS (Lutz 2016), resulting in:

- *Over-activation of the sympathetic nervous system (SNS) or fight/flight response.* The SNS is linked to the "fight or flight" response. Trauma survivors often experience heightened sympathetic arousal. Mind-body movement practices should aim to regulate sympathetic activation through slow, rhythmic movements and grounding exercises, allowing individuals to modulate their stress responses.

- *Under-activation of the ventral vagal complex (VVC), or rest/ digest/social engagement system.* The VVC system is associated with a state of safety, connection, and social engagement. Mind-body movements that promote a sense of safety, such as gentle and repetitive yoga postures (to help cultivate familiarity, expectations, and strengthening progressions), mindful breathing, and non-threatening postures, can help individuals access and activate their VVC system, reducing feelings of threat and anxiety. Interweaving mindfulness and movement can enhance body awareness and help individuals stay present in the moment, while fostering a sense of safety and connection with the present experience. A trauma-informed approach acknowledges the potential triggers and sensitivities associated with trauma. Instructors and practitioners should prioritize creating a safe and supportive environment, offering choices, and allowing individuals to have a sense of control over their practice. The vagus nerve plays a crucial role in regulating the breath (Miller *et al.* 2023). Practices that emphasize breath regulation, such as diaphragmatic breathing or coherent breathing, can influence the ANS, promoting a calm and regulated state.

- *Unpredictable activation of the dorsal vagal complex (DVC) or freeze response.* The dorsal vagal system is associated with immobilization and shutdown responses. Trauma survivors may have challenges with dissociation or feelings of numbness. Mind-body movements that gently engage the body, promote grounding, and provide a sense of agency can help individuals navigate toward a more regulated state. Gradual exposure to different movement patterns and postures, coupled with mindful awareness, allows trauma survivors to build a tolerance to sensations and movements. This progressive approach helps prevent overwhelm and supports the gradual regulation of the nervous system.

By incorporating polyvagal theory into trauma-sensitive mind-body movement practices, individuals can experience a safe and regulated environment that promotes healing (Lutz 2016). Practitioners and therapists specializing in trauma-informed care can guide individuals through these practices, tailoring them to each person's unique needs and preferences.

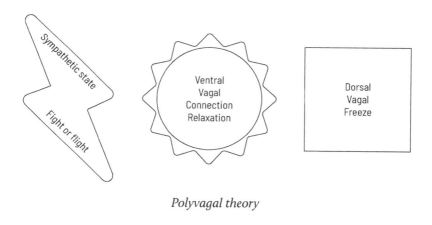

Polyvagal theory

Panchamaya kosha model from yoga philosophy

According to yoga philosophy we are holistic, multidimensional beings, comprised of five distinct yet interactive layers. In this yogic theoretical framework called the panchamaya kosha model, these layers are referred to as the five sheaths of our being or the five koshas. Starting from the outermost layer (the physical body) and moving inward toward the core, each interdependent layer increases in subtlety (Desikchar 1999; Lad 1990).

A yoga therapy practice begins to integrate the outermost koshic layer, using awareness through the senses and in movement via yoga asanas, or physical postures, to the second layer, the energy body, by using yogic breathing or pranayama (Feurstein 2011). As the yoga student begins to understand the flow of vital energy between these two layers, this understanding, in turn, leads to a greater sense of self-understanding and to the interrelations of the underlying mental-emotional and wisdom layers. For example, depression presents with a slouched posture and drooping head, resulting in shallow, restrained breathing and diminished mood in the mental-emotional third layer. Practicing yoga postures or shapes can improve symptoms of depression as the yoga postures replace the posture of depression, and breathing practices can energize the body and mind (Lad 1990; Iyengar 2012). Yoga practices experienced as effective for depression can positively affect intrinsic motivation for continued consistent practice. A consistent, dedicated practice begins to replace the detrimental, subconscious habits of the mind and body with new, healthy habits which continue to lead the practitioner toward a lifelong journey of self-study, self-regulation, and self-realization. Overall, according to the kosha model, though yoga is a comprehensive practice for body and mind, it is ultimately a spiritual practice, and yoga therapy, applied through a trauma-sensitive lens, helps the practitioner to remove the obstacles on his/her/their unique journey to tap into the deepest subtle layer, the spiritual body, leading to the true Self (Sullivan & Robertson 2020; Iyengar 2012). Here freedom to be our true Self means that we can freely live the deeper purpose of our lives.

How to use the panchamaya kosha model in yoga and other mind-body practices

- Use the senses to connect to the physical body or layer, and to the present moment, realizing there is safety *here* and *now*.

- Use breath to connect to the energy body or layer, becoming more self-aware of how to modulate (calm or energize) by using breath control.

- Use the awareness of the above two layers to tap into the emotional body or layer, in order to dampen the effect of the hypervigilant mind from thinking that past traumas belong to the present moment.

- Connect to gut or heart sensations to tap into the wisdom of the intellectual body and to support confidence in decision making and self-advocacy.

- Develop self-trust by cultivating self-regulation to reaffirm trust in the Self, which in essence is connecting the small self to the big Self (one's Source), seeing the Source or Divinity in oneself.

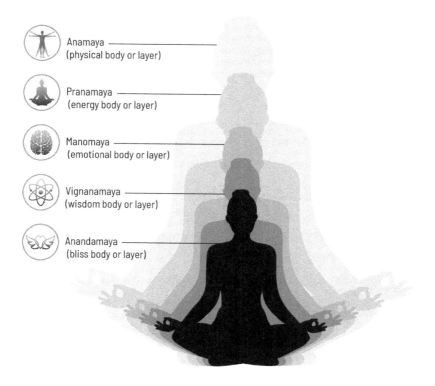

Anamaya
(physical body or layer)

Pranamaya
(energy body or layer)

Manomaya
(emotional body or layer)

Vignanamaya
(wisdom body or layer)

Anandamaya
(bliss body or layer)

Gunas model from Ayurveda

The gunas, as described in Ayurveda, represent three fundamental qualities or energies that influence the mind, body, and consciousness. These qualities are sattva (harmony, purity), rajas (activity, passion), and tamas (inertia, darkness). The gunas model can be applied to promote balance and well-being by addressing various aspects of an individual's experience:

- *Sattva (harmony, purity)*: Sattva represents qualities of balance, clarity, and purity. Practices that cultivate sattva, such as meditation, mindfulness, and gentle yoga, create a calm and focused state of mind, fostering emotional balance and supporting the processing of traumatic experiences.

- *Rajas (activity, passion)*: While rajas can bring energy and passion, an excess of rajasic qualities may lead to restlessness and heightened arousal, which can be challenging for trauma survivors. Mindful movement practices, such as gentle yoga or walking meditation, can help regulate energy associated with rajas, like hypervigilance. It's important to avoid overly stimulating practices that may exacerbate anxiety.

- *Tamas (inertia, darkness)*: Tamas, when excessive, can manifest as lethargy, depression, or a sense of inertia. Gentle movement, breathwork, and practices that promote a sense of grounding can help alleviate tamas. Ayurvedic practices, such as abhyanga (self-massage) with warm oil, may also be used to balance tamas and promote relaxation.

Applying the gunas model to support trauma healing involves creating a therapeutic environment and lifestyle that cultivates sattva, minimizes excess rajas, and addresses imbalances related to tamas. Here are some ways the gunas model may be integrated:

- *Mindful awareness*: Cultivating sattva through mindfulness practices helps individuals become aware of their thoughts, emotions, and bodily sensations without judgment, fostering a sense of clarity and balance.

- *Balanced lifestyle*: Ayurvedic principles can guide individuals toward a balanced lifestyle, including a nourishing diet, regular sleep patterns, and daily routines that promote overall well-being.

- *Yoga and breathwork*: Selecting yoga practices and breathwork techniques that align with an individual's current state of balance and imbalance in the gunas can be beneficial. This may involve adapting the intensity and focus of the practices to the person's needs.

- *Self-care practices*: Ayurvedic self-care practices, such as warm baths, herbal teas, and soothing rituals, can be incorporated to promote relaxation and balance the gunas.

Through the gunas model, Ayurveda provides a holistic framework that considers the individual's constitution, imbalances, and current state of mind and body. Tailoring these practices to the unique needs and preferences of each person under the guidance of qualified Ayurvedic practitioners or healthcare professionals is essential in trauma-informed care (Lutz 2016; Sullivan *et al.* 2018).

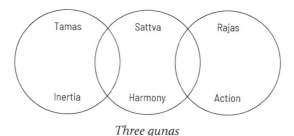

Three gunas

Contemporary neuroscience and ancient yoga philosophy

Polyvagal theory and the gunas

The findings of contemporary neuroscience use polyvagal theory (PVT) to help us understand what happens in the three parts of the ANS while experiencing trauma. Ancient yoga philosophy provides a theory from the context of the panchamaya kosha model (or koshas) and the three gunas as found in the *Samkhya Karika*, the *Bhagavad Gita*, and the *Yoga Sutras of Patanjali*. The gunas are used in the study and application of Ayurvedic, which strives to acknowledge the unique aspects of each individual.

Two additional states: safe mobilization and safe immobilization

Understanding these theories is not just limited to states of danger/threat, but also to times when we need to activate, energize, and focus in order to enjoy the present moment. This includes:

- *safe mobilization*, which is seen as a combination of VVC/SNS activation, or sattvic/rajasic states, in play, enjoyable physical activity, hatha yoga (asana with breath awareness), dance, etc.

- *safe immobilization*, which is a combination of VVC/DVS activation, or sattvic/tamasic states, in nursing/nurturing a baby, intimacy, and active/caring listening, etc. (Sullivan *et al.* 2018).

In summary, the three complexes of the ANS have a parallel in ancient yoga philosophy from the kosha model and in Ayurveda from the gunas model. Following a Western therapeutic perspective, yoga therapy aims to balance the ANS while, from the ancient yogic perspective, yoga therapy aims to balance the gunas while guiding the spiritual journey of self-actualization. Mind-body movement research is now recognized in medical and social sciences, professional organizations, and other governing organizations, bridging the gap between evidence-based and traditional practices to deliver highly effective and easily applicable models to modern complementary and alternative health services. Professionally, this will edify and increase receptivity to the use of many mind-body modalities in the applied sciences, for both preventative and therapeutic integration, especially for building resilience and fostering post-traumatic growth.

The stress response, effect on breath

The stress response is a set of biopsychosocial responses to trauma and to perceived trauma (Burchfield 1979). This includes the release of stress hormones, like cortisol and adrenaline, which can result in increased heart rate, increased respiratory rate, and changes in blood flow to support the body's responses (Russell & Lightman 2019).

The stress response can have significant effects on breathing due to its influence on the ANS, particularly the SNS's "fight or flight" mechanism. When the body experiences stress, whether from physical trauma, emotional stress, or other factors, like perceived stress, it triggers a cascade of physiological responses that can impact all systems of the body (Chu *et al.* 2024). Our focus in this section is the respiratory system. These responses are often subconscious, and some are beyond our control, part of how the brain and body respond for survival from the more primitive parts of our human brain. As we begin to know our tendencies for trauma reactivity, especially those responses we can control, we can begin to use specific pranayamas, the fourth of Patanjali's eight limbs of yoga, in cultivating strategies for self-regulation. Understanding the specifics of how the stress response affects breathing can help us appreciate the intricacies of our human design and guide our choices.

During stress, SNS activation stimulates the respiratory centers in the brain, leading to a variety of possible responses involving altered normal rhythms of breathing (Courtney 2009, Tipton *et al.* 2017; Miller *et al.* 2023). These responses include:

- *Increase in the rate and depth of breathing, known as tachypnea.* Increasing oxygen intake supports the body's increased demand for O_2 for a "fight or flight" response. As the body's oxygen demand increases to support heightened metabolic activity, this may cause the sensation of needing to breathe more deeply or "air hunger" (Tipton *et al.* 2017).

- *Shallow breathing*, due to tension in the chest muscles, resulting in rapid, upper chest breathing. Shallow breathing limits the full expansion of the lungs and can reduce oxygen exchange efficiency. Guiding someone with this tendency to take a deep breath may cause even more constriction and a possible panicked response.

- *Hyperventilation, rapid or deep breathing.* This is common with acute stress or anxiety and can lead to a decrease in carbon dioxide levels in the blood (hypocapnia). The imbalance of O_2 to CO_2 can cause dizziness, tingling and numbing sensations, and confusion.

- *Irregular patterns of rapid breathing followed by brief pauses or irregular intervals between breaths* can also be experienced.

The release of stress hormones like adrenaline, can also cause bronchial smooth muscle contraction and can lead to a constriction of the airways, or bronchoconstriction, making breathing generally more difficult. It is also a common feature of conditions, like asthma or chronic obstructive pulmonary disease (COPD), also known to be exacerbated by stress. Stress-related inflammation and immune system changes can worsen these conditions over time.

Stress and tension can also affect the diaphragm, the primary muscle involved in breathing. Increased muscle tension, particularly in the neck and shoulders, can restrict diaphragmatic movement.

This limits the effectiveness of diaphragmatic breathing, which is deeper and more efficient than chest breathing (Miller *et al.* 2023).

Prolonged or chronic stress may lead to muscle fatigue, including the respiratory muscles. Fatigued respiratory muscles may not function optimally, leading to feelings of breathlessness or difficulty sustaining deep breaths. In some individuals, stress can trigger panic attacks characterized by sudden and intense feelings of fear or anxiety. Panic attacks often involve rapid breathing, chest tightness, and a sense of impending doom. These episodes can further exacerbate respiratory symptoms and increase feelings of distress (Goddard 2017). Breath is the great integrator of multiple body systems, modulating the nervous system via connections between the diaphragm, vagus nerve, fascia, brain, and core muscles (Miller *et al.* 2023).

Management and coping strategies

Pranayama: The yogic practice of pranayama, or breath control, is often referred to as "breathing exercises" in the West. There are hundreds of such techniques used as standalone practices or interwoven with asana, meditation, and relaxation. Some are used for improving focus, calming, building lung capacity, energizing, etc., all of which support an ultimate effect of yoga: refining awareness. For example, diaphragmatic breathing can counteract shallow breathing patterns and promote relaxation. Once the individual has calmed their mind and reduced reactivity to the stressor, restoring calm and steady breathing may take some experimenting with pranayama. Learning a variety of pranayamas can offer choice and facilitate learning to trust one's body.

- *1:1 breathing*, whereby the inhalations and exhalations are evenly smooth, steady, and paced, is an easy start.

- *1:2 breathing* (inhale for 1 count, exhale for 2 counts) can up-regulate the parasympathetic nervous system (PNS), to restore homeostasis (restore elevated heart rate, blood pressure, digestive processes, and other hypervigilant responses).

- *Diaphragmatic breathing* restores the natural rhythm and relationship of lung expansion (chest freely rising/falling) and relaxed abdomen (diaphragm moving in direct response to chest), and indirectly relaxes neck and shoulder muscles. This pranayama is especially useful because it is easy to guide/teach nonverbally and very effective. Placing one hand on the belly and one at the heart helps to understand the tandem movement of these two areas of the body in response to the breath cycle. Practicing diaphragmatic breathing will help undo the tendency of shallow chest breathing, which is typical of the stress response and can become habitual over time. Mind-body awareness here can begin to change that habit, supporting self-regulation.

- *Alternate nostril breathing* is used to balance the right and left hemisphere activity of the brain, and is very effective in calming the nervous system. It can be taught very simply in a nonverbal manner, with gesturing to show the hand placement, indicating inhalation and exhalation, leaving space for students to build their own exploration.

- *Bumblebee breath* is used to calm tension headaches and guide focus on body sensations (physical body vibration and the sense of hearing). Additionally, the effect of vibration is very healing. To practice bumblebee breath, sit comfortably and place the thumbs over the ears. This subconsciously guides tuning into the body. Place the little fingers alongside the nasal flares (not occluding) and allow the other fingers to rest along the sides of the bridge of the nose to the brow, resting gently over a lowered gaze. With each breath, practice slow steady inhalation while humming during exhalation. Children especially enjoy this breath practice. When practiced as a group, each person is breathing/humming at their own pace and the overlap of the humming creates a steady vibration, an effect which tends to be enjoyed by all. In trauma-sensitive yoga, one can choose to participate or not, yet it is rewarding to see how those who do not participate initially begin to enjoy the benefit of the vibrational effects.

- *Lion's breath* is an effective pranayama to support relaxation. To practice this breath, inhale deeply and upon exhalation, stick out your tongue as you say, "HhhAAaaahh," or roar like a lion. This helps to release pent-up tension and/or to express oneself. Often, this can be coupled with shrugging the shoulders on inhalation and dropping the shoulders and sticking out the tongue on exhalation.

- *Four corners breathing* is used to help refine focusing skills and calm the mind. This breath practice is recommended when students are ready to build on the previous pranayamas mentioned here. This breath practice may be more appropriate for those who have conversational English skills and will lend to language learning, building trust in one's body and with the teacher/yoga therapist, and in self-regulation. To practice, spend an equal amount of time in each "corner" of the breath cycle: inhalation, retention, exhalation, retention. Introduce a low count of 1:1:1:1. Repeat for a few cycles, giving time for tuning in, lung expansion/warm up, and becoming familiar with the pace. Gradually add a higher count, 2:2:2:2, 3:3:3:3, and return to 1:1:1:1, while staying comfortable with the pace and pattern. In trauma-sensitive yoga it is not recommended to hold the breath for a long time, hence keep this light. The self-regulation comes from recognizing breath-holding in trigger responses, thus adjusting the breath to disrupt patterns of hypervigilance. This breath practice can be empowering!

Mindfulness and meditation: Practices that focus on present moment awareness can help reduce stress and regulate breathing. Guiding a felt sense of safety in the present moment and using the senses for present moment awareness can be an effective way to learn self-regulation.

Physical activity: Regular exercise can improve general health and resilience, reduce overall stress levels, and improve respiratory function.

Stress reduction techniques found in mind-body modalities: yoga, tai chi, progressive muscle relaxation, eye movement desensitization and reprocessing (EMDR), and biofeedback are just a few.

Professional help: Seeking "top-down" therapy for stress management can provide coping strategies and support. Seeking "bottom-up" therapy can introduce self-regulation tools.

"Top-down" and "bottom-up" are terms known and used in the trauma-informed world, professionally and clinically. Originally, top-down approaches, or psychotherapy, were a more established way to heal and treat trauma. In recent years, bottom-up approaches using mind-body modalities have become incorporated and used as standalone means for guiding inner-resourcing; they're also effective self-regulation tools for trauma healing and related work. This has been due, in large part, to the introduction by Stephen Porges of polyvagal theory (PVT) and an exponential growth of research in recent decades that has followed (Porges 2011). PVT research explores the path and intricate relationships of the vagus nerve, explaining how 80% of nerves between the body and brain are "efferent," giving feedback from the body's sense receptors to the brain (Porges 2022). Research in bottom-up approaches has illuminated how learning to tune into the body is not only effective but necessary for post-traumatic growth (Van der Kolk 2014). Using a bottom-up approach has been shown to be very effective with or without a top-down approach.

Understanding the effects of stress on breathing is important for promoting overall respiratory health, as breath defines life. Using specific breathing techniques is an effective and accessible tool for managing and mitigating the effects of stress-related symptoms, whether acute or chronic. Using various tools from yoga to facilitate self-regulation becomes unique to each person's journey toward healing from trauma and empowering agency in all aspects of life.

Nonverbal communication in teaching trauma-informed yoga

Communication is a key element in any teacher-student role. Verbal communication is only one facet of effective communication. Movement itself is a universal language, one that transcends linguistic boundaries, culture, gender, age, era, and more. In teaching yoga to immigrants and refugees, the presence of a language barrier can indeed present challenges. Being prepared to comfortably lead a yoga practice with nonverbal communication can have several advantages. Making time to study and become trauma-informed and trauma-aware of the biopsychosocial and spiritual mechanisms of human responses is foundational. Another key is to be prepared within the context of one's profession. Last, doing research to learn about the population you wish to serve is necessary for creating best practices using yoga for trauma healing.

These include:

- Giving space for people to shift their focus from listening to more specific movement cues to taking in the somatic experience of the practice. While recognized for centuries in traditional yoga, the way self-realization results from consistent yoga practice has become a present-day focus in the research world. The capacity to connect the sensations of the body to the felt sense of safety in present moment awareness begins to shift reactive tendencies into reflective habits. While this is an ideal outcome for all yogis, it is a cultivated skill unique to each person and does not necessarily need direction from language communication.

- Avoiding a rushed pace will help the student relax around exploring movement and breath. This also allows more time for the teacher to observe and, therefore, assess what can be better tailored to help the student.

- The teacher can take cues from the student's ability to follow the intended practice, and, in real time, respond to the student's physical abilities and emotional capacity. The teacher can readjust to introduce "safe" movement to ensure a sense of feeling successful in practicing yoga. This helps the students connect to and trust their bodies, especially their inner strength. There is the potential when working this way to create a felt sense of collaboration within the shared practice.

- Both the teacher and student(s) will refine how to use gestures to communicate through continued experience of a shared practice.

- Building familiarity with each other from the repeated yoga practice gives an opportunity to eventually introduce language learning: sharing the names of colors, movements, body parts, natural surroundings, etc. Healing comes from hearing each person's voice. From yoga philosophy we understand that stagnated energy accumulates in the fifth or throat chakra, when one is not "heard," when they feel that their voice doesn't matter and/or is not respected. From the perspective of polyvagal theory, leading with a warm smile and non-threatening body language initiates a vagal brake, up-regulating PNS responses. Therefore, beginning to use language in meaningful ways contributes to healing from trauma, without having to formally bring attention to the process.

Creating a relationship of trust from feeling seen and heard can come from just one practice, and amplifies the processes listed above.

To effectively manage nonverbal communication where language is a barrier, consider the following strategies:

- *Demonstration*: Prioritize slow, steady, simple, and accessible demonstrations of yoga poses, preparations, and sequences. Use your own body to show the general alignment and movement patterns, allowing students to visually observe you and mimic your actions. Because students' initial focus is on imitating the teacher, the ultimate challenge becomes guiding the student to explore and tailor the practice on their own by tapping into their own physical, mental, and emotional bodies.

- *Visual aids*: Use visual aids, such as erase boards, flip charts, books, posters, sequence handouts, or instructional videos that illustrate yoga poses and their names. This can help reinforce understanding and provide a reference point for students to follow along and for home practice.

- *Avoid hands-on adjustments*: The first premise of yoga is ahimsa, to do no harm, so we do not want to contribute to trauma triggers, which can easily come from encroaching on personal space or from physical touch, even when the intention is gentle hands-on adjustments to guide students into proper alignment during poses. While physical touch can be a powerful means of communication, conveying support and encouragement (even in the absence of verbal instruction), if we cannot ask for consent and respect personal boundaries, we would be acting unethically to assume permission in applying touch. Unless the teacher is licensed in a trauma-responsive modality, it would be outside scope of practice to do otherwise.

- *Use of props*: Incorporate yoga props, such as blocks, straps, blankets, and bolsters, to assist students in achieving "support and safety," not necessarily correct alignment, and deepen their practice. Demonstrating how to use props effectively can enhance understanding without the need for verbal explanation.

- *Body language*: Pay careful attention to your own body language and facial expressions. Maintain a warm and open demeanor, conveying empathy, encouragement, and enthusiasm through your nonverbal cues. Smiling, nodding, and making eye contact can help foster a sense of being "seen" as well as of connection and trust with your students.

- *Slow paced instruction*: Break down instructions into simple, manageable steps and deliver them at a slow and steady pace. Allow sufficient time for students to observe, process, and execute each movement before transitioning to the next.

- *Repetition and reinforcement*: Repeat key movements multiple times throughout the class to reinforce learning. Comfort comes from knowing what to expect, thus practice means building familiarity with movement. Encourage students to follow along with each repetition, gradually building progressions from familiarity and therefore building self-confidence with the poses.

- *Encourage observation*: Encourage students to observe and learn from their peers. Create an opportunity for a student to "shine" by demonstrating. By creating a supportive and collaborative atmosphere, students can glean insights from each other's movements and adjustments, enhancing their understanding and learning experience. This helps to develop confidence and may support building agency in the long run.

- *Encourage feedback*: Foster open communication by inviting students to provide feedback on their experience. Nonverbal cues, such as nodding, thumbs up, or hand gestures can be used to signal understanding or express concerns or preferences.

• *Cultural sensitivity*: Be mindful of cultural differences and sensitivities that may influence students' responses to nonverbal cues. Respect cultural norms regarding physical contact, personal space, and communication styles, adapting your approach, as needed, to ensure inclusivity and cultural sensitivity. This means taking time to educate yourself on the cultural background and immediate situation of the students.

• As a teacher/leader, make time to *tune in to yourself*, be reflective. Relax, let go of any agenda, convey the essence of what you prepared to teach, but don't worry about the details. Be yourself! Enjoy that you will learn and receive much more than you intend to give.

• *Trust the yoga and trust your intuition* for being intentional and taking time to prepare.

By incorporating these strategies into your teaching approach, you can effectively manage nonverbal communication in yoga classes in any population/setting. With immigrants, refugees, and asylum seekers, these points will facilitate creating an inclusive and accessible learning environment, where movement serves as a universal language of connection and healing, from the collective group experience to the development of each individual's yogic tools for self-regulation.

Sequence theme: Releasing emotions (Estimated teaching time is 30 minutes)

Seated on the floor, on a block/blanket/prop

Props: Mat, blanket, block (substitute what is available for any of the props)

This sequence is illustrated in photos on the pages immediately following the steps below.

1. Easy pose: one hand at heart, one hand at belly, attention to breath

    a. Twist

    b. Side bend

    c. Cat/cow while seated with hands on knees

2. Low lunge

3. Reverse warrior l

4. Powerful (Chair)

5. Goddess

6. Triangle

7. Deep squat

8. Cradle

9. Knee down twist

10. Corpse: With the following options using the prop from #1

    a. Prop under knees

    b. Support under head

    c. Blanket over body

For #1, adding a side bend, twist and cat/cow from sitting in easy pose will provide a subtle warm up to include all the actions of the spine, providing a gentle transition into the sequence for all other shapes and movements. This gives the yoga instructor a chance to observe to accommodate any special needs by adding or omitting different poses or shapes in the remaining sequence.

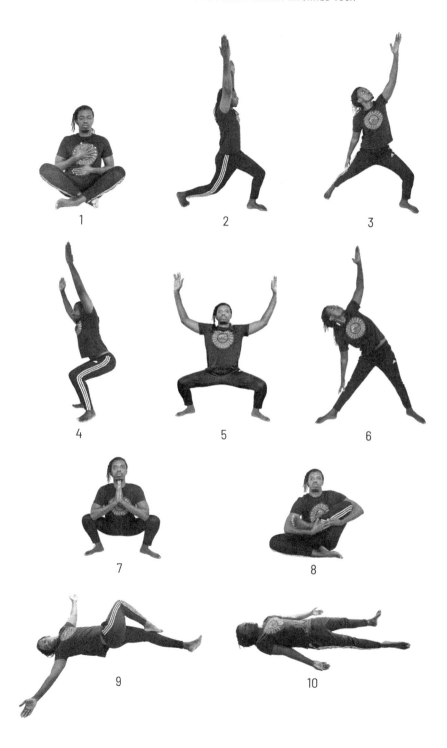

Mona and her journey to serve refugees

Mona Hilbawi Flynn was born in Damascus, Syria, and immigrated to the US with her parents (father Syrian and mother Iraqi) and younger sister, at age 4. Due to the Gulf War and the Syrian Crisis, many of her family members now live all over the world. Unable to travel back to Iraq or Syria, or see her extended family easily, Mona now advocates for immigrants and refugees where she lives in Greensboro, North Carolina.

Owner of Life Fit Yoga, she is seasoned in mind-body practices, with over 35 years in exercise physiology and teaching, blending preventive and rehabilitative therapies. Understanding the challenges of resettlement firsthand, and the potential of offering yoga for well-being, Mona founded The Yoga Connection, a 501c3 (a nonprofit designation by the US federal government) which aims to provide empowerment and community to immigrant and refugee women through a group yoga therapy class.

Through recent doctoral studies she created, and now offers, an evidence-based certificate-bearing course, Trauma-Sensitive Training for Mind-Body Professionals, with modules focused on the immigrant population. Mona is a hatha yoga teacher with an Iyengar influence, Yoga Alliance E-RYT500/YACEP, a C-IAYT with the International Association of Yoga Therapists (IAYT), and a TRE (Trauma and Tension Releasing Exercise) Advanced Provider.

> As yoga guides us to practice awareness, acceptance, abhyasa (perseverance), and ahimsa (doing no harm) while removing the obstacles for living our dharma, may we apply those guiding principles to helping others on their journey too. Hope and healing comes when we realize that we are all One, on the same journey essentially. Enrichment comes from embracing those who cross our paths.

As a first-generation Syrian American woman, my family immigrated to this country when I was 4 years old, my father aiming to provide his daughters opportunities and freedoms of the American Dream.

His teaching career fell short, as a heart condition turned into a failed open-heart surgery and several strokes cascaded his health situation. Though our mom was a certified math teacher, her training was not recognized in the United States, so she became the breadwinner of the family over many years of tedious sewing. Watching my mother lead provided an awareness of the strength and survival skills of women, especially immigrant women. In meeting other immigrant women over the years, I am constantly intrigued by the interplay of unique events, opportunities, and personalities toward settlement outcomes.

Our parents invoked a sense of empowerment through education and work ethic. My college education prepared me to be an exercise physiologist with knowledge to serve a wide range of "special populations" (for example, high risk pregnancies, severe osteoporosis, fibromyalgia, etc.), applying the benefits of physical activity to many dimensions of health. Connections provided me with initial great jobs in my field, and eventually Life Fit, Inc. was born, a business oriented around using movement to empower "living."

In 2019, Life Fit students, local teachers, and friends locked arms for a shared seva, supporting successful resettlement while providing yoga to immigrant and refugee women in a program called "Yoga Therapy for Immigrant & Refugee Women." Three years later, despite the pandemic, the program evolved to become The Yoga Connection (TYC), a 501c3 with an active board, consistent volunteers, and collaborative community partners. TYC now incorporates an evidence-based, required trauma-informed training for all volunteers and a trauma-sensitive training for TYC teachers.

In the infinite ways to develop, sequence, and facilitate a yoga practice with and for others, being authentic and seeing the unique needs of each person and situation are the keys. The above yoga sequence incorporates a trauma-sensitive approach which includes considerations for planning and guiding yoga for immigrants and refugees. The lessons come from my experiences in the five-year TYC program for immigrant and refugee women, a program which continues to evolve successfully from the collaborative efforts of many compassionate people, an enriching space where I continue to learn.

The program has two mission statements:

- The Yoga Connection (TYC) builds community for immigrant and refugee women in Guilford County and supports their well-being and empowerment.

- TYC provides service opportunities for yoga therapists and teachers, college students, and community members.

and two vision statements:

- TYC envisions providing for the resettlement of immigrant and refugee women, their well-being through yoga practice, and their connection to the broader community.

- In addition, area college students can benefit from internships with TYC, and local yoga instructors can work toward certification and continuing education in yoga therapy.

The program is shaped by each person who arrives to each eight-week session, bringing their perspective, whether a participant who recently arrived to the United States, or a volunteer. What I have noticed is how those who return not only show up for themselves on their mat, but for each other. This is the ultimate gift of radical acceptance and shared humanity.

Sequencing toward peak poses is not important at TYC. Instead, the focus is more on holistic classes that are safe and brave spaces, accessible, welcoming, and empowering for all who arrive to join: the participants, volunteers, and teachers. To support the ideals of trauma-sensitive yoga for immigrant and refugee women, all volunteers complete trauma-informed training and yoga teachers complete a trauma-sensitive training, provided for them. Classes are set up in a circle, and the classroom has several exit doors and windows with natural light. Teachers use simple and welcoming language, guide sense awareness and calming pranayamas to cultivate self-regulation and present moment awareness, show respect, offer choice, and prioritize the importance of hearing each person's voice.

Welcome exercise: The yoga instructor chooses one word as the mantra and theme for the class, for example, "love." While many cultures and languages are present in each class, participants are invited to introduce themselves as best they can in every class and contribute to a class conversation by sharing where they are from, translating the word into their home language, and the volunteers add an offering of synonyms, like "kindness," "compassion," "support." This practice invites choice and collaboration, and builds respect and empowerment. Additionally, it becomes not only a unique and significant way for building language skills, but a relaxed way to guide an immediate felt sense of community within each class.

As I wrote my contribution for this book, I was completing research for my doctoral dissertation, "Impact of a Community Yoga Therapy Program on Well-being for Immigrant and Refugee Women." The mixed methods study assessed a community-based, trauma-sensitive yoga program for immigrant and refugee women, using three different scales and a current qualitative method (Sort and Sift, Think and Shift), to understand improvements in three domains of well-being—physical, mental/emotional, and social health—from the perspective of the participants. The results suggest that such programs can support successful acculturation and improve physical and mental health, language skills, and social bonding, serving as a framework for enhancing healthcare equity and quality of life for this population. I am excited to continue sharing the findings and recommendations from my study in future workshops and trainings, along with mentoring replication of programs in communities worldwide.

The content of this book shares our experiences in meeting the needs of the immigrants, refugees, and asylum seekers in communities we felt drawn to serve. We hope to meet you as we create future offerings that will bridge the content here for professional development, continuing education, and collaborative efforts for innovative change, welcoming our "new neighbors" in our One World.

CHAPTER 2

Practical Guidance in Sharing Trauma-Informed Yoga

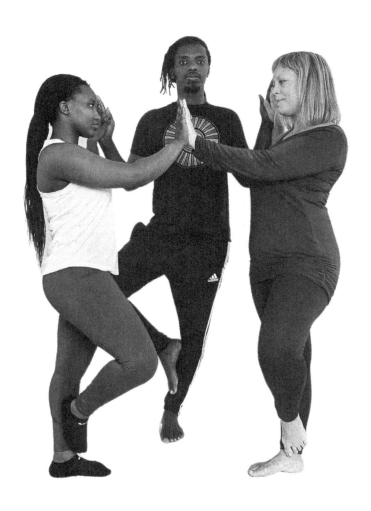

The window of tolerance

While working with clients who may have experienced trauma on their immigration journeys, be aware of their "window of tolerance." This is where information can be learned and new habits can be formed. We want to meet our clients in this window.

As explained below, the psychology-based understanding of the window of tolerance very much resembles the yoga therapy models presented by Mona Flynn in Chapter 1; another example of how yoga meets science.

When noticing signs of hyperarousal—anxiety, shaking, crying, screaming—or hypoarousal—distracted, numb, flat, or disengaged— it's helpful to guide the client toward finding something to help them come back into their window of tolerance. The techniques described below can expand one's window of tolerance. The client may become more aware when they are becoming dysregulated. Your job, as a trauma-informed yoga therapist, is to notice when something you are doing may be taking them out of that window. Adjust your practice to help the client stay in their window of tolerance by using these trauma-informed techniques.

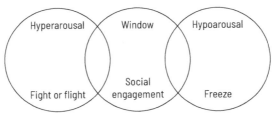

Window of tolerance

Signs of trauma release

- cold or hot

- trembling

- crying

- holding breath

- disassociating (disconnecting from the body and present moment)

- screaming

- thrashing arms

- difficulty concentrating

Bringing your client back to the present moment

- Invite your clients to feel their feet on the ground, their bottom on the chair, etc.

- Ask your clients to feel their legs, arms, stomach, etc.

- Remind your client that they are safe, and describe the setting.

- Ask if you can touch your client's feet with your feet.

- Ask if you can touch your client's hand.

- Invite your client back into the present moment by asking, for example, "What day is it?" "Where are you?"

IMPORTANT BEST PRACTICE NOTE

If you notice a participant having one of these trauma releases, be present with them. You don't need to be their mental health therapist or say the right thing. Unless you're a trained, licensed, or certified mental health practitioner, this is out of your scope of service. Witnessing is enough. Create a safe space for them to feel their feelings. Try to resist offering a remedy, toy, hug, or tissue. Although it is good to have tissues nearby in case they ask for one. After it appears they have been able to experience that release, you can offer a grounding practice to help them self-regulate.

Although connecting with migrants can be very intimate and social, it is a best practice not to ask participants to share their story with you or for you to ask follow-up questions. If you feel that they want to share this with you or have a therapy-like interaction, thank them for their vulnerability. Afterwards, discuss the possibility of referrals to therapists in the area that they could talk to about this. After a participant or group has an emotional release, use yoga, dance, or a playful art project for integration to shift back into their "window of tolerance." This is a perfect example of *co-regulation*: when your participant regulates their emotions with the support of an individual or group.

Follow-up support with a therapist is not always available for various reasons, like long waits for appointments, while migrants are on the move. For this reason, it's best not to encourage emotional release without proper integration and follow-up. Allow your participants to open up at their own pace. Don't ask too many questions or make any requests.

Note: Taking a deep breath is not always something a client can do when having a trauma release. This is not necessarily a helpful cue.

A QUICK SENSORY GROUNDING TECHNIQUE

5: Acknowledge FIVE things you see around you. It could be a pen, a spot on the ceiling, anything in your surroundings.

4: Acknowledge FOUR things you can touch around you. It could be your hair, a pillow, or the ground under your feet.

3: Acknowledge THREE things you hear. This could be any external sound. If you can hear your belly rumbling that counts! Focus on things you can hear outside of your body.

2: Acknowledge TWO things you can smell. Maybe you are in your office and smell pencil, or maybe you are in your bedroom and smell a pillow. If you need to take a brief walk to find a scent, you could smell soap in your bathroom, or nature outside.

1: Acknowledge ONE thing you can taste. What does the inside of your mouth taste like—gum, coffee, or the sandwich from lunch?

These sensory grounding techniques may help to co-regulate your student or client's emotional state. Walking on the earth can be helpful...walking, moving.

Nonverbal communication

In Chapter 1, contributor Mona Flynn thoroughly discussed her experience practicing nonverbal communication with The Yoga Connection program participants. Often refugee programs can attract refugees from many countries. On the last weekend we served at the border, in February 2024, 17 countries were represented, crossing the Texas/Mexico border in Brownsville, Texas.

Below are a few important techniques we have learned by using nonverbal communication in our Casa de Paz SLV programs.

- *Acknowledge your level of fluency* in the language(s) spoken and adapt to accommodate. Teach nonverbally unless you can communicate clearly.

- Using a *soothing voice/tone* as you guide is a very simple tool that can be incredibly supportive, regardless of the language spoken.

- It is *best to not use cell phones* to translate while teaching or giving sessions, unless absolutely necessary. Write out lessons and vocabulary needed and have that in front of you as you teach. Practice before teaching. As we have all experienced, when a person looks at their phone, we have lost their attention. We don't want this to happen during a class or healing session. It's is best to be fully present.

- Unless you are fluent, you will likely not understand your private client when they are having an emotional release, talking, and crying. It is *best to have an interpreter* with you. Interpreters may not be available at all times. If your interpreter is accustomed to the healing you provide, it can be a beautiful healing partnership.

- *Find other ways to comfort your clients with nonverbal teaching.* For example, nonverbally invite them to tell you about the art they created, by pointing to it, smiling. If you can learn the words for "tell me," that is enough. In Spanish we would say, "Dime por favor..." Short phrases are very accepted in an international setting. Everyone is trying to communicate, and often with limited language skills.

- *Energy healing, acupuncture, acupressure, music, and massage* are very effective nonverbal ways to offer trauma support. Yoga and art can also be shared beautifully in a nonverbal way. There are also welcoming exercises you can do that create a melting pot of contributions in a variety of languages. (See Welcome Exercise in Chapter 1 presented by contributor Mona Flynn.)

Touch and movement positions

Always be aware that asylum seekers may have experienced some form of physical or sexual abuse. For this reason, be very conscious of touch, as well as body positions during movement classes.

Avoid movements that involve bending over and straddles, especially when there are onlookers. When teaching tween and teen girls in the public eye, provide them as much privacy as possible. A private tent or room is best. If you inadvertently display tween and teen girls doing yoga poses they could become prey for human trafficking.

As yogis, let's remember that contemporary yoga movement originated as a form of exercise and stretching to teach teen boys to be able to meditate. It was also, and still is, practiced in the privacy of one's home as a personal self-care practice. Many learned yoga privately from relatives. It was rarely done in mixed gender groups.

That is a Western adaptation of yoga. Many yoga poses can feel very vulnerable when practiced in groups. I have had enough clients tell me they couldn't learn yoga in a group because they would get too emotional, releasing uncontrollable tears. This does not happen to everyone, but yoga does have the power to touch us deeply when in a safe setting. Some poses can activate trauma and emotions locked within the somatic body tissue.

Regarding touch, it's best practice to not offer hands-on assists. Always ask permission before putting your hands on your client. Avoid the chest and pelvic areas. Comfort can be provided by touching shoulders, hands, and feet with permission.

Multicultural sensitivity and awareness

My personal journey with privilege

When I was 19, I wanted to join the Peace Corp. This felt like a calling at the time. The Peace Corp knew better. They saw I needed experience working in the developing world and that it would also be helpful to be somewhat fluent in the language. It wasn't until I was in my 40s, and after receiving a Masters in International Administration from World Learning, Inc., that I was financially able to live in such countries on my own. I received my yoga teaching certificate at Nosara Institute in Nosara, Costa Rica, in 2004. Like so many of my cohorts who stayed on or traveled to neighboring countries, I decided to live there for four more months. I had just sold my house and had some savings.

I taught yoga in the jungle at a local cafe by the beach that had a beautiful wood floor. It was during this time that I learned *so* much about my privilege. The locals quickly checked my privilege. I had to be friendly and polite. Ticos are very polite and humble. They saw people from the US as "arrogant."

I needed to speak Spanish and I learned to live in rough conditions.

No air conditioning in temperatures that hovered around 90 degrees Fahrenheit daily (32 degrees Celcius). No car. I walked and took buses like the locals. I learned how to deal with the "cat calls" and how to protect my belongings when traveling. I learned to make reservations at youth hostels with limited Spanish, and to navigate all the requests for my money. Showers were often cold. Sometimes I had to walk through mud and trash dumps. It was through my experiences teaching yoga and providing healing arts in developing countries, such as Costa Rica, Jamaica, and Panama, that I became prepared to work with migrants.

In my Master's degree program, I learned a great deal about multicultural awareness and sensitivity. This training gave me the knowledge I needed to work in developing countries. However, it was the lived experiences that really taught me what I needed to know.

In Panama, there were a lot of indigenous people, so I was able to experience that culture with its mix of missionary influence.

In Jamaica, I learned about the economic inequities that led to a certain attitude toward white people as colonizers and exploiters.

I did my best to understand the locals and live with the locals. The more I met them where they were, the more I was accepted. But not as family. I was never accepted as family. That was made clear to me directly by some of my coworkers and friends. "You are not one of us."

At World Learning, Inc., it was emphasized by all my professors and cohorts from all over the world that the people who should be doing service work are the people from that country and/or community. For this reason it is a best practice to provide trainings of trainers, designed to train the people in the community to teach trauma-informed yoga. These trainings are created with the input of the community. What do they need? When Casa de Paz SLV did an online survey of our service community, it showed that the community wanted to learn English. Based on this input, we include English as a second language exercises in all our offerings. With that said, it is helpful for your service community to experience the benefits of yoga, so they have a context to provide input.

Often, the mothers were so grateful for a moment of peace while we entertained their children and they received body work or did yoga. The children enjoyed a healthy distraction from the horrors of their immigration journey. Parents appreciated what they considered "childcare." We shared art and yoga for babies, toddlers, and preschool age children as well. We soon learned that this was a need and to always make it available in our programs.

Things to know about privilege

- Learn from the locals. How do they live? How do they survive?

- Do not expect to be served. You are there to serve. Learn how to be of service, how to make a contribution rather than taking away an experience.

- Learn how to teach yoga without props. Sometimes, the best teaching experiences happen on the street, in someone's home, tent, or on the beach. Can you teach yoga effectively and safely without props? If not, learn how.

  During the pandemic, our clients, usually families, were quarantining in tents. We created YouTube practice videos with this in mind. Our potential clients were living in small, multigenerational spaces. Know those you serve and how they live each day, including what they have access to. Do they even have internet access, and if so, when? Some encampments provide wifi only at certain times of the day, or migrants or refugees need to pay to use it.

- It is best to not wear expensive clothing or jewelry. You will be less likely to be robbed or seen for the money you can provide.

- For the same reasons, do not make gift-giving visible. You will be seen exclusively as someone who can provide things. This creates dependency rather than self-sufficiency and resilience. Often, there is a way to funnel your money unobtrusively, by purchasing meals that are served to everyone or buying items that are needed and distributed fairly to those who are in the most need.

- Carry your money on your person. If you put down your purse or backpack, it will likely be stolen. Don't get upset if this happens. Own your part in the mistake and try not to repeat it. Some need to repeat this lesson many times before they learn.

- Always travel with a "buddy" (travel companion). Your buddy should be someone you know who has a safe reputation. There are many who pose as helpful, only to take advantage later. Another lesson to be learned. Our volunteers choose a buddy before crossing into Mexico.

- Learn the language. There are apps that can help you. For example, I use Duolingo and SpanishDict. Form a study group. You will learn quickly this way. Immersion helps. Always try to speak the language, even if you didn't take the time to study enough. You will quickly pick up so much more if you try. Refugee camps tend to be international places, so refugees and asylum seekers are used to figuring out what you have to say with sign language and context. You will soon be able to do the same. Communication happens in a variety of ways. Using your phone for translation can take away from your connection experience and I discourage it. Only use it if you have no other choice and communication is not coming across.

I have provided references about white privilege in the Further Reading section. Take the time to read them and pass them on to your volunteers. White privilege is probably one of the biggest problems in the service field. Coming from countries of wealth, we have the privilege to serve, but we need to check our privilege constantly. If not, it will interfere with the ability to serve.

Camping keeps coming to mind as a helpful skill for migrant work. Do you like to camp? If you don't camp or don't like to camp, you will likely have trouble serving in a refugee camp. Conditions tend to be even worse with poor sanitary conditions. This is often the first thing that is addressed in a refugee camp, but is still not up to US standards. Toilets and showers are shared by hundreds of people. Disease spreads easily. Come prepared with sanitary wipes and your own toilet paper. Wash up well after serving by washing with disinfecting soaps or tea tree oil. Bag up and wash your clothing right away to avoid spreading germs in your home or lodging space. Children (and adults) can carry contagious skin conditions, such as scabies or ringworm.

Ultimately, it is a best practice to pass on what you are providing to the service community with trainings of trainers. This is what we strive for at Casa de Paz SLV. We have board members who are also trainers based at the border of Texas and Mexico and in the Dzaleka Refugee Camp in Malawi, Africa. We have also trained asylum seekers waiting at the border in Sharing Yoga and in Partner and Self Massage. We continue to invite this type of participation in all our programs.

Attract diverse teams that include professionals from the region where you serve. When it feels right, invite some of these professionals to sit on your board or to be part of a core teaching team. Create a board or teaching team that includes people of various ages, those of the global majority, people who identify as LGBTQIA+, and representatives from the communities you serve.

Always engage the community you are serving. Learn about their culture and traditions. How much can you blend their ways of living into what you are providing? When I shared a yoga class series in an indigenous village in Bocas del Toro, Panama, and at the border of Texas and Mexico, we sang the songs of that culture as a "song swap." I taught them a children's song like "head, shoulders, knees and toes" for movement and English as a second language skills development. They taught me the songs they learned in church.

Casa de Paz SLV provides migrants in the encampment and shelters in Mexico with essential oils as sprays and roll-ons, herbal sun tea kits, healthy natural foods, and massage. These are all practices that are done for healthcare in indigenous and rural villages in Central America. We always provide instructions in Spanish with the essential oils and explain how to use them verbally, taking care with those oils that may irritate eyes, like tea tree oil and peppermint. Groups would often gather informally to learn the natural methods together and a more serious discussion about natural medicine would often take place. We receive many donations of essential oils.

We provide instructions for making sun tea, by putting a variety of medicinal teas in a small (8oz) mason jar. Teas might include those for relaxation, immune boosting, or digestion. All are very much needed by asylum seekers while on their immigration journey. The food quality at encampments is poor, and sanitary conditions are not good. Disease spreads easily, and anxiety is high due to the unknown.

Many Central American migrants lean into prayer and faith in God to provide and protect them. Their faith is woven into their daily expressions and conversation. In general, we observe that migrants are more accustomed to natural medicine, so they easily embrace what we provide. However, migrants come from all over the world. You will also come across people who are from developed countries and who are used to western medicine. Offer services that are inviting and welcoming for all and that don't take away from their culture and traditions, but help them to maintain them. They can be a source of comfort.

On that note, many migrants are from the LGBQTIA+ community because, for religious reasons, it is too dangerous for them to be themselves in their home country. They are often not accepted, beaten, killed, and sometimes incarcerated for being queer, where they will likely be killed by their inmates. Asylum is usually granted to these migrants because they are in danger. Those supporting migrants are encouraged to educate themselves about the LGBQ-TIA+ community and how best to be of support. Visit the GLAAD website (www.glaad.org) to learn how to be an ally and offer the best support possible.

CHAPTER 3

Creating a Trauma-Informed Yoga Program

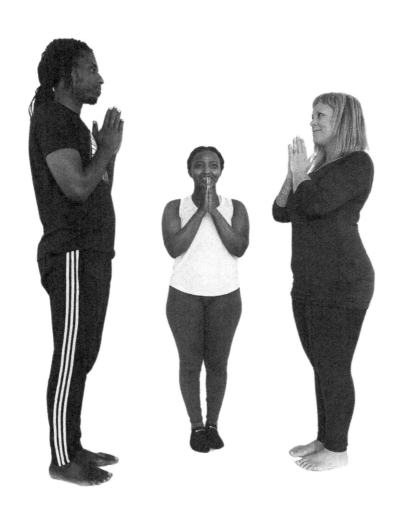

Setting the stage for healing to take place

Inform the service community of what services you are offering, either on a sign and/or verbally at the beginning of the programs. By doing so you are obtaining "implied consent," which is the law for providing healthcare in Mexico. It is imperative that you learn and follow the laws of the locations where you want to serve. Communicate clearly with your nonprofit partners about the services you will be providing, and do your best to follow their policies and procedures. Always remember that you are a guest.

Providing trauma-informed yoga instruction

Because follow-up is not always an option due to marginalization, and because migrants are always on the move, it is best to avoid yoga poses that may reactivate trauma symptoms. Many migrants also come from conservative cultures, and doing certain poses in public can be culturally inappropriate. In this book, we provide sample sequences that are culturally sensitive and avoid trauma reactivation. We avoid sharing yoga poses like down dog, cat/cow, straddles, and happy baby because they resemble sexual positions. Also, offering physical assists can surprise a student who may have experienced physical abuse. Touch may also be culturally inappropriate. Volunteer yoga instructors enjoy figuring out new ways to create similar results, like doing plank rather than downward-facing dog or cat–cow in sun salutations and flexing the spine while seated. Suggest that your clients close their eyes as a choice and not a requirement. Migrants are always on guard for danger. Perhaps it is better not to suggest it at all. Migrants can be so compliant. Create new ways to get the same results.

If a qualified volunteer is doing body work, ask each client for consent. Be sure the therapist is trauma trained, aware of areas of the body that might be reactive, and knows that quick movements could cause a trauma response. Inform clients as you move around them. Something to be aware of: Your service population may be so needy and afraid that they unconsciously act overly compliant, so offering multiple opportunities to decline is a best practice.

If your service is short-term and follow-up mental healthcare is likely limited, instead of providing yoga therapy for trauma practice trauma-informed yoga and simply provide comfort or respite. Form partnerships with local therapists, medical, and mental health providers in your service area, so you can give referrals. Follow the consent practices of the country where you serve, and of the client's culture. It is best to not touch children. If they want a hug, you can hug back, depending on the laws of the country and the protocol of the institution where you serve. Some suggest doing a side-body hug as an emotionally safer practice.

Some practices help integrate challenging emotions that may arise from doing yoga or being in a therapeutic setting. Often, that involves doing playful poses, like rocking in bow pose, or doing free movement to danceable music. The tweens and teens like to do the challenging asana. You can also share poses that create resilience, like warrior pose, boat, and other core strengtheners.

Resilience sequence (Estimated teaching time is 30 min)

This sequence is illustrated in photos on the pages immediately following the steps below.

1. Mountain

2. & 3. Complete breath—inhale shoulders to ears and drop dramatically on exhale at least three times.

4. Step back into lunge.

   • Show modifications with knee on floor, hands on knee, or arms lifted.

5. Step back into plank and hold for 5–8 breaths.

6. Lower down and come into low cobra.

   • Rise up to plank and step back into lunge on opposite side, repeating step 4 above.

7. Come into Warrior II.

   • Optional additions: warrior twist, exalted warrior, and side angle stretch.

8. Starfish standing.

   • Warrior series on other side, repeating step 7 above.

9. Tree on both sides.

   • Optional group tree in circle: Ask participants if they find it easier to do in a group or solo?

10. Come to sitting and into boat—partner boat is also a playful and challenging option to add.

    • Lie on back by dropping arms and legs dramatically with legs apart and arms away from sides.

11. Revolving stomach twist with knees bent on both sides.

12. 10-minute corpse pose.

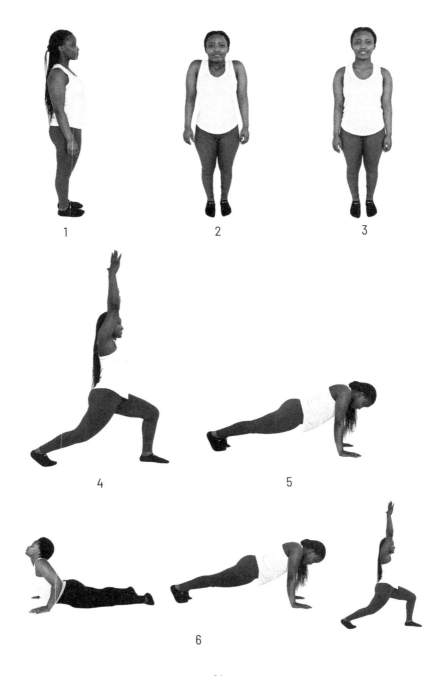

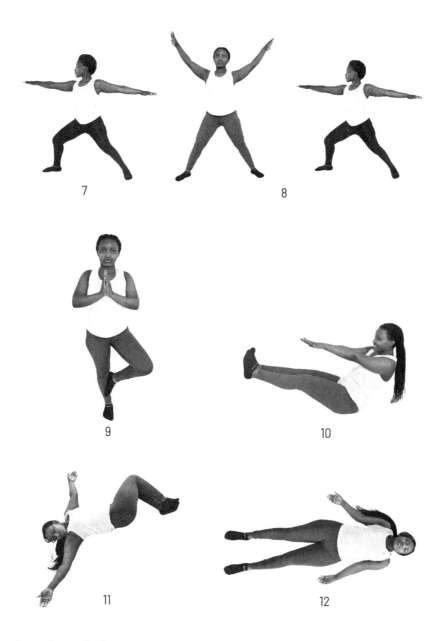

7   8

9   10

11   12

In order to help participants actually learn trauma-informed yoga therapy self-regulation techniques, share poses that you repeat, like a sun salutation class. We also refer clients to the Casa de Paz SLV YouTube channel to continue to practice. They enjoy seeing familiar faces, so it's helpful when service trip volunteers can make follow up videos for your YouTube channel. One of our volunteer yoga instructors made several trauma-informed yoga practice YouTube videos with his partner. When they got married last fall, I posted a photo of their wedding picture on our Facebook page. It was probably one of our most popular posts. Connection is so important to a culture used to having family and community around all the time, even if it is online. This is a form of comfort that can make a huge difference in the mental health of your service community.

Trauma-informed modified sun salutation sequence (Estimated teaching time is 30 min)

This sequence is illustrated in photos on the pages immediately following the steps below.

1. Mountain.

2. Step back to lunge.

3. Step back to plank.

4. Lower down to sphinx.

5. Push up to plank.

6. Step forward to lunge with opposite foot.

7. Step into mountain pose.

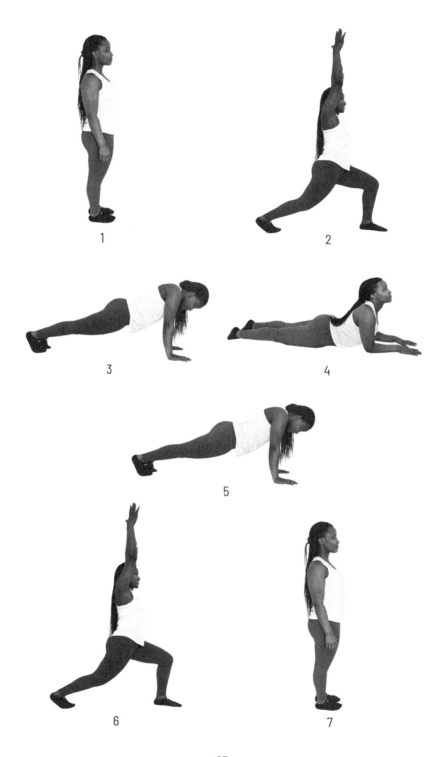

1

2

3

4

5

6

7

In all our Casa de Paz SLV programs, we provide a postcard that has a QR code to our website. From here, our students and clients can find us on social media, where we have a private Facebook group and a YouTube channel for follow-up practices and support. When we have enough volunteer licensed therapists, we have offered free "support chats." This requires a longer-term commitment from your volunteers and an ability to refer out for ongoing therapy.

Guidance for trauma-informed yoga instruction

- Gentle heart openers release grief.

- Gentle hip openers release sexual trauma and old trauma with parents/partners/siblings/abusers.

- Spine stretches are beneficial for overall health and sleeping on the ground.

- Core strengtheners work well at the end to seal energy body openings. They also encourage inner strength.

- Embryo pose (garbasana) is helpful for integration, bringing all awareness and energy inward.

- It's best to go slow and gentle. Open the body slowly, and integrate often. Long savasanas and embryo pose.

- Seated forward bend promotes inward exploration. Can be too reflective for a one-time class.

- Forward bend followed by fish pose may create an emotional release. Grief. There may be a need to vocalize or cry. Only do if follow-up support is available.

- Sound and breath help release emotions. Make space for and encourage sound.

- See "Touch and movement positions" in Chapter 2, regarding touch. Best to use words rather than touch for assists.

- Due to cultural expectations, cisgender men often need a way to release their anger and energy. Share a warrior series, sun salutations, sound, lion's pose/breath, and alternate nostril breathing for calming.

- Young children seem to need to release energy with vigorous movement and short teaching periods (30 minutes, then switch to art therapy or vice versa).

- Vigorous movement and sound release trauma.

- Partner and group yoga poses are very playful for groups. They can lift the mood.

- The culture you are serving may be modest. Instructing women to bend over or straddle their legs to do yoga may not be culturally appropriate. They may giggle or refuse to do the shape if you suggest it accidentally. Create sequences that *do not* include cat/cow, down dog, or big straddles. Even standing forward bends can create some embarrassment. Any pose that resembles a sexual position may reactivate trauma symptoms or may be culturally insensitive. Position women so they are not facing the public or others. A private tent or room is ideal.

- It is best not to encourage big emotional releases with, for example, camel or intense forward bends and then big backbends.

- Teach in a spiritually neutral way. In other words, perhaps avoid chanting "Om" or using Hindu terms. Instead, teach culturally sensitive yoga. For example, you can use the words "light" or "energy," but your participants might understand that better if you also say "God." This may also be confusing because many think God is an old man in heaven. However, some do understand. One time I asked a group, "What do you think light is?" and one student responded, "Peace."

- Focus on providing comfort, relief, and gentle transformation of trauma symptoms.

- Use English words that translate in the most common language spoken, so sun salutation might translate to "sun greeting."

CHAPTER 4

Creating a Program or Nonprofit

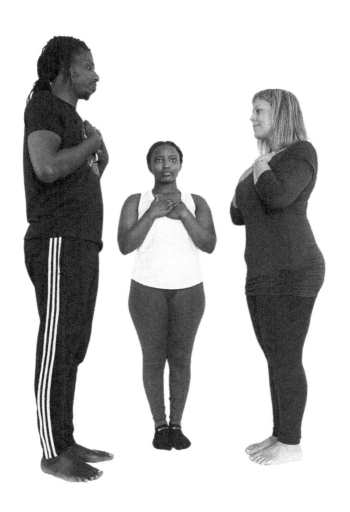

At some point, you may decide you want to create a nonprofit. Below are some factors to consider before you start:

- Your private funding sources have been asked multiple times, and you need to be able to access more funding sources to continue serving.

- Be prepared to create an organization with staff, volunteers, liability forms, insurance coverage, and accountability. Building a nonprofit can take place over many years.

- Receiving grants can require record keeping and evaluations of programs. This takes time. Applying for grants is a full-time job. More established nonprofits have full-time grant writers on staff. Do you have the volunteers or energy to apply for multiple grants? It can take many, many applications before you succeed.

- Do you have the time to create the documents needed for grants? These include board member and staff CVs, a budget, the project scope, logistics (space rental and transportation), and more.

- Do you have an attorney who will help you with liability issues? Highly recommended. You can usually find one who will do it "pro bono" (as a volunteer).

- In the US, being a 501c3 nonprofit is appealing to donors and funders because they can write their donation off on their taxes at the end of the year. This option can attract more donations. For tax purposes, nonprofits need to provide a letter to each donor, acknowledging the donation.

Instructions and forms for becoming a nonprofit are accessible on your government's website. Casa de Paz SLV hired a consultant to walk us through the process. It is also something anyone can figure out. It's not that difficult. You do need a bank account, officers (board members), a physical address, and a mailing address. In order to open a bank account for a nonprofit in the United States, you also need to become a legal business entity in your state.

Recognize that the work of becoming a fundable nonprofit takes time and can be accomplished over many years. Allow yourself this time and, as I learned from my immigrant and border colleagues, "Don't give up."

After careful consideration, you may choose to move forward and become a nonprofit, or you may decide to work with an organization with a similar mission that is already formed. Your program can be supported by their funding, human resources, and established liability protocol.

The administrative tasks of creating a trauma-informed yoga program

Find nonprofit partners who are already serving in your target area. Find out what they are doing. Help them, then show them what you would like to share. I suggest being upfront with your skill set and area of expertise, so there are no misunderstandings. Other organizations to partner with may include churches, as well as nonprofits with a similar mission. Churches have large followings and often have shelters or community programs that are serving your population. They are always looking for volunteers and new programs.

Nonprofits that may be serving in your service area are Doctors without Borders, Save the Children, United Way, and other less widely known groups helping to serve food, provide basic needs, and offer education. Find out who the "gatekeepers" are and set up a "meet and greet." Volunteer, learn from that experience, and talk to those in charge while you help out. Find out if anyone else is providing mental health support or yoga. You will not want to duplicate efforts. People can be very territorial about their projects, and some feel a sense of competition for limited funding—even yoga teachers, who often struggle to piece together a livelihood. Enlist their support by sharing with them how your program is different along with the benefits it provides.

Create a website and/or social media account where you can show photos and videos of trauma-informed yoga programs that have been successful. Be sure the images include the population you plan to serve. It is essential to be very respectful when taking photos. Ask permission. Explain why the photo is needed. Take photos from the back of your subject(s) or block out the eyes of all those in the image with the edit feature on your phone or computer. Asylum seekers are often fleeing dangerous situations and it is not helpful to publicize their location. Children are not an exception.

It is wise to have photo releases in longer-term programs. In my opinion, when migrants are traveling, asking them to sign release forms is not a trauma-sensitive practice. Any release forms used need to be translated in the language of those who are signing, so they are understood.

Create a YouTube channel to share trauma-informed yoga practices. This can be very helpful once your clients have immigrated, are living in a more isolated situation, and need practices they can do at home on their own. Many migrants do not own computers and phone use charges add up. Keep the videos short for this reason. Always check your privilege and remember that new immigrants are often living with family members and sharing technology for school, work, or doing the paperwork involved in acquiring citizenship. They are also very busy with survival issues, like working long, hard hours and raising children.

Create an online support program where asylum seekers, refugees, and new immigrants can do phone or Zoom calls with a licensed or certified practitioner. At Casa de Paz SLV, only licensed social workers and therapists facilitate these calls. Trauma-informed yoga therapists with experience in mental health may also do these with care and follow up. We support the client until they feel a sense of completion. After about six sessions, we refer them to a free therapist in their area. Our volunteer staff is limited, so this is the best way to conserve our resources. It's also valuable for our clients to be able to access ongoing mental health resources in their area. Many are dealing with PTSD, anxiety, and depression and need ongoing care.

Create a private Facebook group for posting your new YouTube practices and offering a "safer" (not secure or confidential…it's Facebook) forum for discussion and questions. Asylum seekers quickly learn to be very careful about sharing personal details on social media. However, some still crave the community and participate cautiously. Some have shared religious or inspirational songs. Music is a universal self-regulation tool.

Create a sustainable program that will continue when you leave. This takes time. Find yoga therapists and trauma-informed yoga instructors in your service area; those who live there and interact with the immigrant community. There are many children of first-generation immigrants living along borders. Some may not be trained in trauma-informed yoga, so you may need to provide training and supervision. We have found that these yoga instructors need to be paid. They are living in a marginalized community themselves. Find ways to pay them with donations and grants. Research what the average yoga teacher is paid in the service area and pay that rate. When you can't pay the going rate, then recognize them as volunteers who are being paid a "stipend." Casa de Paz SLV started paying $25-an-hour stipends. An issue that arises is that this level of pay is not a living wage, so turnover of these volunteers is frequent. With recent inflation, we are now paying our teachers $35/hour as a stipend. Project Coordinator receives a $40/hr stipend (2024).

Translate all written materials on your website and your eblasts in the languages most commonly spoken by your participants. You may find volunteers who will do this for you. It can be more difficult to find translators for indigenous languages, but it is often needed.

Organizing, vetting, and onboarding volunteers

Organizing and onboarding volunteers is time consuming, but is often needed to facilitate an underfunded program. It is also attractive to funders to see what the nonprofit is contributing in terms of in-kind service. "In-kind" means donated time or items. Be sure to track all your in-kind contributions, including volunteer time.

Creating an online presence with a website and social media helps to get the word out to attract volunteers. Networking with other nonprofits informed about what you are offering can provide referrals.

Vetting volunteers

We are working with mental health issues and complex trauma. It is wise for volunteers to go through a thorough interview and trauma-informed training process, as well as training in how to help people to self- or co-regulate. It is helpful to accept only volunteers who are already trained in this way and are certified and licensed in their professions; most should be bilingual. Check references. This is how you will make a final decision about an applicant. It is not recommended to skip this step or to accept volunteers simply based on a professional, verbal referral. Try to get at least three references. You will likely get two calls back. Aim for consistency in responses. Reference-check questions to ask include:

- Is this person reliable?

- Are they trustworthy?

- Are they able to handle stressful situations?

- How?

- Do they work well independently and with a team?

As you conduct service trips, certain leadership approaches will provide smooth teamwork and solidify the group. More relaxed leadership styles may cause problems. When in a high-stress and high-risk environment, it is most helpful for all involved that everything flows smoothly. When a service trip is not running smoothly because of team member personal issues, everyone is affected. You may choose to fine-tune your approach and policies when this happens.

Some suggest volunteers receive a background check. For short-term volunteering, this step is often skipped. There are online services that provide background checks for a small fee. Check with your legal support to see what your nonprofit or program needs to protect it from liability issues.

Liability waiver for volunteers

Create a liability waiver for your volunteers. Have an attorney draw this up for you. Be sure the risks are explained in this waiver and that you have a copy before service takes place. Do not skip this. Unfortunately, liability is a huge issue in many developed countries. People sue. People can get hurt or be negligent. If you have a nonprofit, your board members will be liable. If you don't, you will be liable. Protect yourself and your board members.

Onboarding volunteers

Very quickly, you will find the need for a training manual and/or video and training topics to discuss or share. You will also want to create a volunteer application, Frequently Asked Questions (FAQs), and interview questions. Because Casa de Paz SLV serves in a high-risk area, we also require all volunteers to sign a liability waiver, which was created by a team of volunteer attorneys.

Invite the board of directors and your nonprofit leaders with experience serving to help with interviewing and training volunteers. They provide volunteers with different perspectives about the service you are providing. It's always good to have leadership representation from the area where you are serving. Keep the interview and training under an hour. Respect that everyone is volunteering and that their time is valuable. Meeting on Zoom allows for a certain level of confidentiality and international participation. Learning the time zone differences of your members and volunteers is helpful. Choose times that work for everyone present.

Some key features of a training manual and/or video

Describe the service area in an honest way, so volunteers know exactly what they are volunteering to do. Explain any risks up front.

Visit www.casadepazslv.org/volunteer for an example of our very thorough volunteer application. It has been updated many times and has now been designed for all volunteer opportunities. It includes our nonprofit volunteer policies and a detailed description of all the tasks that volunteering can involve. I suggest you request volunteer applications, training manuals, and videos from various and similar organizations and adopt the policies that fit your mission. If you borrow language you should obtain permission from the nonprofit that created it.

Casa de Paz SLV also provides a FAQ handout for volunteers attending service trips. Our volunteers receive this after their references have been checked. We provide this handout with the liability waiver. Signing the liability waiver indicates their commitment to the service trip. We also ask for their signed commitment in the volunteer application, so we usually have no problem with volunteers leaving mid-service trip or no shows.

Casa de Paz SLV has adopted *The Four Agreements* as a tool for creating harmony as a volunteer team. We ask our volunteers to familiarize themselves with these agreements and to do their best to follow them. We find that harmony does ensue when these agreements are followed by our volunteer teams. We put a big emphasis on refraining from gossip, as gossip can be a form of entertainment in certain cultures. We all know how harmful gossip can be. Not gossiping takes some self-discipline and is a learning journey.

THE FOUR AGREEMENTS
by Don Miguel Ruiz (2021)

Be impeccable with your word

Speak with integrity. Say only what you mean. Avoid using the word to speak against yourself or to gossip about others. Use the power of your word in the direction of truth and love.

Don't take anything personally

Nothing others do is because of you. What others say and do is a projection of their own reality, their own dream. When you are immune to the opinions and actions of others, you won't be the victim of needless suffering.

Don't make assumptions

Find the courage to ask questions and express what you really want. Communicate with others as clearly as you can to avoid misunderstandings, sadness, and drama. With just this one agreement, you can completely transform your life.

Always do your best

Your best is going to change from moment to moment; it will be different when you are healthy as opposed to sick. Under any circumstance, simply do your best, and you will avoid self-judgment, self-abuse, and regret.

Centering

Before all meetings and serving, we center. This is something that is never skipped. It is a way to come into the present moment after driving and unpacking supplies for serving. It is also a way to connect and co-regulate as a team and create a unified purpose or vision for your day. On Casa de Paz SLV service trips, volunteers take turns leading centering. Examples might include a grounding exercise, a moment of silence, or sharing three Oms.

Days off and activities

I highly recommend taking days off between service days. This allows volunteers to reset and come back to themselves after very intense service. Suggest activities that are going on in the area. Take an excursion or go on an outing together. Attend a Spanish class. Some choose to work on their days off. On our service trips, we discourage that, but can't always control it. If volunteers choose to work on their days off, request that they be rested and present to serve.

Sometimes it can be tempting for volunteers to party. They may choose to go to Mexico for their day off and drink margaritas. This is always fun, but you can tell who drank the day before they returned to serve. Those volunteers are often not able to serve at their best. I would discourage these types of excursions, as they can be tiring and leave volunteers in a state where they are not able to serve at their best. Instead, suggest that volunteers go to easy-to-attend events that are close to where everyone stays. If volunteers want to have longer excursions and party experiences, you can suggest they extend their trip for that type of travel play.

Handling donations

It's good for your volunteers to know in advance that material donations are distributed fairly, based on need. To distribute in this way, we usually give donations to the person in the leadership role at each center where we serve.

You will find that some people just don't like fundraising. For this reason, it is always a good idea to give your volunteers opportunities to donate a minimum amount instead. For Casa de Paz SLV service trips, we have asked for $500 toward administrative costs and supplies. Volunteers also have to cover their own travel and lodging, so we try to make this affordable. Other nonprofits may ask for much more, and that amount might include donations to the communities where you serve.

Debriefing

Debriefing is often required by funders when working with mental health and in high-risk areas. This can be done while walking and/

or driving back to your vehicles or lodging. You may also share meals before, during, and/or after serving. Check in about anything volunteers want to share. Sharing usually happens naturally because volunteers want to discuss their experience. Often there are things that are witnessed that break our hearts. We do our best to hold confidentiality, while also sharing some of the emotions that surface while serving. If you have future plans to serve together, this can also be a time to discuss the best ways to serve next time. It's important to process the trauma you are witnessing. Follow-up processing may be needed with your support group or therapist. If that is needed, I suggest volunteers seek that support when they return home. We ask that all volunteers have a self-care practice to process emotions as they arise during the service trip. Self-care and self-regulation techniques utilized form an important interview question, and should be included in your volunteer training.

Flexibility

I can't emphasize this enough. Aside from checking one's privilege, this is probably the most important quality needed when working in a border or refugee camp setting. As hard as you try, communication gets lost and details can be misunderstood. Meetings may not happen as planned and your volunteer team may need to adjust. It is important to make sure that your volunteers and staff are aware of this and do not have expectations that everything will flow smoothly or as planned.

Confidentiality

If your volunteers are not licensed mental health practitioners, they may not have experience with holding confidentiality. This may be something you need to train them in and model. Even when discussing participants as a team, it is best to hold confidentiality and speak in general about any concerns.

Training of trainers model

Training the community you serve to continue to self-regulate their trauma symptoms is a best practice in the international service field. It is more effective and sustainable than dropping in, doing a program, or providing a service and leaving. In long-term stay settings, like refugee camps, some organizations have trained refugees to be yoga instructors. Program sustainability is a basic requirement for most funding.

At Casa de Paz SLV, we have done four different trainings of trainers over the past five years: Share Yoga for all ages and unaccompanied minors; Partner and Self Massage for adults; a Trauma-Informed Training for "case workers"; and we have hired and trained teachers in our service area.

Share Yoga

Since we were not going to be present indefinitely, we have offered Share Yoga. This program teaches students a modified sun salutation and there is an opportunity for question and answer. The graduates are invited to co-teach, by modeling the poses alongside the trained instructors. This training attracted men, women, and teens.

At a government shelter during the pandemic, we offered a four-week online Share Yoga for the teens. Up to three classes (groups of approximately 20 students) of unaccompanied minors attended each time. We repeated poses and had a check-in after each class to see how the yoga affected the teens and if they had any questions. At the end, we encouraged them to become yoga teachers if they wanted. This was considered a vocational program to expose the teens to a job they could do when they leave the shelter.

Partner and Self Massage

We did this program with teens, men, and women. The instruction was translated and a handout was provided. Partner massage was taught in a trauma-informed way and could be done sitting in a chair. Self-massage was based in Chinese medicine and lymphatic massage.

Trauma-Informed Training of "case workers"

At the Dzaleka Refugee Camp we partner with MUTU.org, a group of volunteer "case workers" who process emotions with the arts. First, the Casa de Paz SLV board of directors met with some of the families via Zoom to hear their heartbreaking stories. We listened and they appreciated that we cared. We invited them to share a song to help co-regulate the emotions that surfaced. We all sang and they drummed and danced. Everything had to be translated by our board member and the director of MUTU.org. Although English classes are offered in the refugee camp, the primary language spoken is Swahili. The Dzaleka refugees feel so forgotten and without hope that suicide rates are high. The "case workers" are often the first responders to suicides, so the training was also designed to support them. Our board chair and licensed social worker, who works with refugees in the US full time, provided the training online. They had technical issues because the refugees at the camp have to pay for their own internet, so we would often run out of time.

What we have learned serving in Dzaleka is that it is not possible for our US nonprofit to send money overseas. It is best to work with a nonprofit foundation whose primary role is to grant funding to other nonprofits like ours. Additional steps are required of US nonprofit foundations to donate to international nonprofits. To date we have not been able to provide the needed funding to continue programs there. At a minimum, we need internet access and to pay for a TV. Our trainings were done on a laptop for a large group to view. We are welcome to do service trips there, but costs are high to travel to Africa from the United States. Our board member from the camp will be settling in the United States soon, and hopefully we can do more once he gets here.

Hire and train teachers in your service location

With a generous grant from a Colorado-based fine artist, Casa de Paz SLV hired two trauma-informed and experienced facilitators who live at the border of Texas and Mexico. They specialize in trauma-informed yoga and therapeutic art for marginalized populations in their community. They are native to the US border with Mexico and bilingual. These instructors have also been trauma trained by Casa de Paz SLV. Our first two-day beach retreat for 20 unaccompanied minor teens took place in April 2024. A one-day retreat for 15 unaccompanied minor teen girls took place in November 2024. With future funding, we hope to continue this program for more unaccompanied minor teens.

Funding your program

When your program and/or service population is trending in the media daily you will attract large sums from private donors. This money can be raised via Facebook/Instagram fundraisers, GoFundMe, art auction donations, fundraising events, like dinners, donation-based yoga classes, concerts or dances, webinars, and by expanding your reach with new volunteers helping with outreach.

Community-based funding is often not sustainable. Instead, you may choose to form a nonprofit and apply for grants. There is a great deal of federal (US government) money available for mental health and immigration relief. Federal grants require a lot of paperwork. Finding private foundations is encouraged. This takes a team effort at the beginning, until you can hire staff for this purpose. Knowing your funders personally helps. Invite funders to visit your program to volunteer or observe. Getting media coverage and having a website with images and videos of your service will help attract funders. You will need letters of support from the community you serve when applying for grants.

When serving in marginalized communities, I have learned many lessons from those who I serve. When I really tune into their struggles and how they navigate their challenges, I witness resilience, unwavering faith, and the strength to never give up. I would have stopped doing this work much sooner if it wasn't for these teachings because of the many obstacles I experienced attempting to provide this service. They keep me going even today. The lessons I learn from migrants and first-generation immigrants living at the border have helped me, as a white woman of privilege, to remain committed to keeping Casa de Paz SLV alive and thriving. Partnering with the unaccompanied-minor, US-wide government shelter system, and our many other partners at the border, we are always needing to adjust to more conservative policies and liability concerns. Many of these organizations have strict guidelines that we are not accustomed to operating within. We do it for the children we serve. We know their lives are better because of what we share with them.

Nonprofits rely solely on donations and grants. Volunteers are one way to expand your reach (network of donors) by inviting their community to your GoFundMe, Facebook fundraiser, and other events, via newsletter and in-person outreach. It is helpful to ask your volunteers to gather donations (or discounts) for your service supplies and any items on your Amazon wish list. You can also invite them to host a fundraiser in their community on behalf of the nonprofit or program you are providing. Many come forward with their own unique ideas. Be sure to always update your volunteers on how their efforts are helping, and be sure to thank them often.

Building a base of support for matching and in-kind donations becomes important as you apply to larger funding sources, like foundations and the federal government. Ongoing fundraising campaigns for specific projects help to build this support and funding base.

FUNDRAISING IDEAS

- Some volunteers may be part of other nonprofits that will make donations.

- Some donors will make larger end-of-year donations of as much as $500 or more. It helps to be a nonprofit, so they can write these larger donations off on their annual taxes. End-of-year giving is very common for this purpose (US practice).

- Invite donors to send monthly checks as "patrons."

- Ask yoga studio owners to offer donation-based classes for your organization, or have a donation jar in their studio.

- Make holiday or note cards from a series of paintings of your service community, or art made by them, and sell these over the holidays, during the giving season.

- Request donations of supplies, such as basic needs, healthy snacks, aromatherapy, and yoga mats. Each spring, the Give Back Yoga Foundation offers an annual mat grant for seva projects.

- Create an Amazon wish list, where your supporters can donate basic-needs items, art, and healing arts supplies. Many choose this option versus sending money. They feel their money will go directly to migrants.

- Find corporate sponsors for end-of-year donations. Knowing people who work for the corporation who can advocate for your cause is critical. It's all about who you know. Invite sponsors to match donations. Use giving season donations and other fundraising campaigns for specific programs.

- Meet with your state representative. Find out their stance on immigration. If they are supportive, stay in touch. Request a letter of support. This will make all the difference in receiving federal funding.

- Create a fundraising event or educational webinar that you can offer yearly as your annual fundraiser. Your organization will soon become known for this event, and interest and donations will build.

- Evaluate all fundraising efforts and problem solve those that are not generating donations any longer. Try something new.

CHAPTER 5

Serving in an Immigrant/ Refugee Setting

Collaborating within Your Unique Community

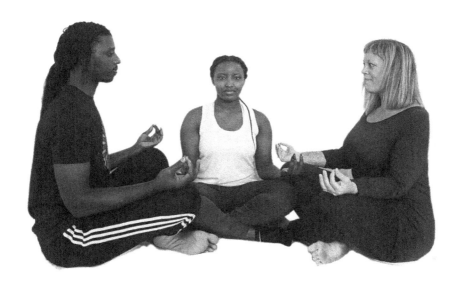

Who are the gatekeepers in your service community?

Find out. Approach them humbly with your credentials, resources, and assistance. Often, they will need to learn the benefits of yoga, so be prepared to share that. Not until we started providing yoga to hundreds of children, out in the open in the sidewalk schools, did the benefits of yoga become apparent. Don't assume everyone knows. They don't. I would go so far as to say that yoga and other holistic practices are considered taboo in certain religions.

Before we were able to start sharing yoga classes, Casa de Paz SLV was encouraged to buy meals for thousands and to donate camping supplies, hygiene items, and clothing. Do not come empty-handed and take away an experience. This is not about having a personal experience to check off your bucket list. You are serving the most vulnerable, and it is important to take this role seriously and to come prepared.

Spend time with the gatekeepers. Serve in the way they do. Serve, listen, and learn. Even though it's not yoga, you are being interviewed. You are also receiving training. It's a valuable opportunity to see how it's done in the area you want to serve.

Gatekeepers look like missionaries, nonprofits providing respite (often churches), organizations that provide food, like World Kitchen, and nonprofits providing medical care, like Doctors without Borders.

Most of the gatekeepers are from religious organizations, so it is important to be accepting of organized religion. Come to an understanding within yourself about aligning with religious organizations. Some provide service better than others. Some offer it unconditionally. Others are more culturally insensitive and seeking new members for their church.

Migrants learn how to work the system and many go along for the respite they receive, even if the religion is not their faith. Decide which organizations have a similar service approach and philosophy. In my experience, it's best not to compromise around this. If you partner with an organization that does not have the same values, you may end up in awkward situations as you serve.

While serving at the border, I have trained our volunteer yoga teachers not to Om, to respect others religions. One of our yoga teachers did it anyway. It became our calling card. On the next service trip, I emphasized not to Om. In the sidewalk school where we served, one of the lead teachers asked, "Why don't I hear the children Oming? I told him why and he said, "We are not like that. We love hearing the Om."

What informed my decision not to Om was based on a previous experience I had serving in an indigenous village in Panama. We Omed and the children shared their church songs. Soon the village pastor came around and sent a scolding look at the children. They all backed away from me. I asked why and one of the youngest and most enlightened of the group looked at the pastor and said, "We can't." It all depends on where you are serving. You need to ask yourself, what is more important, chanting Om or being able to continue sharing yoga as "fitness?" That is how they saw yoga in this village. Whether it is seen as fitness or not, the healing benefits are the same, and that is what really matters. If even one of those children kept doing yoga for the rest of their life, I know I made a difference. I am one of those kids who learned yoga in high school and did it for the rest of my life.

Which type of seva is right for you?

If working internationally in rougher conditions or running a non-profit feels overwhelming, you have options. Create what works for you and what you have time to accomplish in a professional way. If you don't feel like you have adequate experience and don't want to acquire it, there are other ways to serve from the comfort of a developed country. You can serve in a nearby city that has an influx of refugees. This is what they do at The Yoga Connection in Greensboro, North Carolina, USA. Mona Flynn describes their program in more detail in Chapter 1. When serving in these settings it is important to be multiculturally sensitive and sensitive to the lived experience of refugees, asylum seekers, and new immigrants. Be aware of their complex trauma history, their immigration journey, and the challenges that come with assimilating to a new culture and living with very few resources.

References

Barrett, R. (2023) *Casa de Paz SLV Volunteer Training Manual.*

Burchfield, S.R. (1979) "The stress response: a new perspective." *Psychosomatic Medicine*, 41(8), 661–672.

Caperchione, C.M., Kolt, G.S., & Mummery, W.K. (2009) "Physical activity in culturally and linguistically diverse migrant groups to Western society: a review of barriers, enablers, and experiences." *Sports Medicine,* 39(3), 167–177.

Centers for Disease Control and Prevention: National Center for Injury Prevention and Control. (2024) *About Mental Health.* www.cdc.gov/mentalhealth/learn/index.htm.

Chu B., Marwaha K., Sanvictores T., Awosika, A.O., *et al.* (2022) "Physiology, stress reaction." In: *StatPearls* [Internet]. Treasure Island, FL: StatPearls Publishing. www.ncbi.nlm.nih.gov/books/NBK541120.

Courtney, R. (2009) "The functions of breathing and its dysfunctions and their relationship to breathing therapy." *International Journal of Osteopathic Medicine*, 12(3), 78–85.

Desikachar, T.V.K. (1999) *The Heart of Yoga.* Rochester, VT: Inner Traditions International.

Feuerstein, G. (2011) *Encyclopedia of Yoga and Tantra.* Boston: Shambhala Publications.

Global Migration Data Analysis Centre (2024) *Forced Migration or Displacement.* Migration Data Portal. www.migrationdataportal.org/themes/forced-migration-or-displacement.

Goddard A.W. (2017) "The neurobiology of panic: a chronic stress disorder." *Chronic Stress.* https://doi.org/10.1177/2470547017736038.

International Organization for Migration. (2022) *World Migration Report.* https://worldmigrationreport.iom.int/wmr-2022-interactive.

Iyengar, B.K.S. (2012) *Core of the Yoga Sutras: The Definitive Guide to the Philosophy of Yoga.* New York: Harper Thorsons.

Kumar, G.S., Soffer, G., & Begg, D. (2021) "Movement-based therapies for resettled refugee populations in the United States." *International Journal of Yoga Therapy*, 31(1).

Lad, V. (1990) *Ayurveda: The Science of Self-Healing: A Practical Guide* (2nd ed.). Twin Lakes, WI: Lotus Press.

Lutz, J. (2016, February) "Classical yoga postures." In *Proceedings of the Yoga & Psyche Conference (2014)*. Newcastle upon Tyne: Cambridge Scholars Publishing, p.103.

Miller, J., Cordoza, G., Santos, A., San Juan, E., & Olimpo, C. (2023) *Body by Breath: The Science and Practice of Physical and Emotional Resilience*. Las Vegas: Victory Belt Publishing.

Mitchell, K.S., Dick, A.M., DiMartino, D.M., Smith, B., *et al.* (2014) "A pilot study of a randomized controlled trial of yoga as an intervention for PTSD symptoms in women." *Journal of Traumatic Stress*, 27(2), 121–128.

Müller, M., Khamis, D., Srivastava, D., Exadaktylos, A.K., *et al.* (2018) "Understanding refugees' health." *Seminars in Neurology*, 38(2), 152–162.

Nickerson, A., Bryant, R.A., Silove, D., & Steel, Z. (2011) "A critical review of psychological treatments of posttraumatic stress disorder in refugees." *Clinical Psychology Review*, 31(3), 399–417.

Porges, S.W. (2011) *The Polyvagal Theory: Neurophysiological Foundations of Emotions, Attachment, Communication, and Self-Regulation* (Norton series on interpersonal neurobiology). New York: WW Norton & Company.

Porges, S.W. (2022) "Polyvagal theory: a science of safety." *Frontiers in Integrative Neuroscience*, 16.

Reed, R. (2022) "Four lines." *Art Love Lifestyle Magazine*, Spring. www.magcloud.com/webviewer/2241469.

Refugee Health Technical Assistance Center (2024) *Mental Health*. www.refugee-healthta.org/physical-mental-health/mental-health/index.html.

Ruiz, M. (2021) *The Four Agreements: A Practical Guide to Personal Freedom* (17th ed.). San Rafael: Amber-Allen Publishing.

Russell, G., & Lightman, S. (2019) "The human stress response." *National Reviews Endocrinology*, 15, 525–534.

Sengupta, P. (2012) "Health impacts of yoga and pranayama: a state-of-the-art review." *International Journal of Preventive Medicine*, 3(7), 444–458.

Sullivan, M.B., & Robertson, L.C.H. (2020) *Understanding Yoga Therapy: Applied Philosophy and Science for Health and Well-Being*. New York: Routledge.

Sullivan, M.B., Erb, M., Schmalzl, L., Moonaz, S., *et al.* (2018) "Yoga therapy and polyvagal theory: the convergence of traditional wisdom and contemporary neuroscience for self-regulation and resilience." *Frontiers in Human Neuroscience*, 12, 329–370.

Tipton, M.J., Harper, A., Paton, J.F., & Costello, J.T. (2017) 'The human ventilatory response to stress: rate or depth?' *The Journal of Physiology*, 595(17), 5729–5752.

US Department of State: Bureau of Population, Refugees, and Migration (n.d.) *Admissions & Arrivals*. Refugee Processing Center. www.wrapsnet.org/admissions-and-arrivals.

Van der Kolk, B. (2014) *The Body Keeps the Score: Brain, Mind, and Body in the Healing of Trauma*. New York: Penguin.

Wegnelius, C.J., & Petersson, E. (2018) "Cultural background and societal influence on coping strategies for physical activity among immigrant women." *Journal of Transcultural Nursing*, 29(1), 54–63.

Westgard, B., Martinson, B.C., Maciosek, M., Brown, M., *et al.* (2021) "Prevalence of cardiovascular disease and risk factors among Somali immigrants and refugees." *Journal of Immigrant and Minority Health*, 23(4), 680–688.

Wieland, M.L., Weis, J.A., Palmer, T., Goodson, M., *et al.* (2012) "Physical activity and nutrition among immigrant and refugee women: a community based participatory research approach." *Women's Health Issues*, 22(2), 225–232.

World Health Organization (n.d.) *Mental Health.* www.who.int/health-topics/mental-health#tab=tab_2.

Further Reading

Collins, C. (2018) "What white privilege really is." *Learning for Justice*, 60. www.learningforjustice.org/magazine/fall-2018/what-is-white-privilege-really.

GLAAD (2024) *Tips for Allies of Transgender People.* www.glaad.org/transgender/allies.

Lyons, S. (2019) *The Repair of Early Trauma: A "Bottom Up" Approach.* Beacon House. https://chosen.care/the-repair-of-early-trauma-a-bottom-up-approach.

Waldman, K. (2018) "A sociologist examines the white fragility that prevents white Americans from confronting racism." *The New Yorker.* www.newyorker.com/books/page-turner/a-sociologist-examines-the-white-fragility-that-prevents-white-americans-from-confronting-racism.

Author Biographies

Author

Gina M. Barrett, MIA, C- IAYT, E-RYT200 is an author and trauma-informed yoga therapist in the Phoenix Rising Yoga Therapy tradition, specializing in sexual assault trauma and sex re-education. With a Master's degree in International Administration, she has worked for many years in the nonprofit social justice and environmental fields. In 2019, she founded Casa de Paz San Luis Valley (SLV), based in Crestone, Colorado, USA, with a mission to provide holistic trauma support for asylum seekers, refugees, and new immigrants internationally. Gina was the recipient of the 2022 International Association of Yoga Therapist Seva Award for creating trauma-informed yoga programs at the border of Texas and Mexico. In her private practice, Eastern and Somatic Therapies, Gina shares Phoenix Rising Yoga Therapy, professional development trainings, private therapeutic movement instruction (yoga and qigong), sacred sexuality, wellness, and equine therapy retreats. Gina summers at her cabin in her native state of Conway, Massachusetts, USA. To learn more about Gina, her services, workshops, trainings, and other books, visit www.ginambarrett.com.

Contributor

Mona L.H. Flynn, EdD, C-IAYT, E-RYT500, YACEP, TRE Advanced Provider, was born in Damascus, Syria, and now advocates for immigrants and refugees from where she currently lives in Greensboro, North Carolina. Owner of Life Fit Yoga, she is seasoned in mind-body practices, with over 35 years in exercise physiology and yoga, blending preventive and rehabilitative therapies. Understanding the challenges of resettlement firsthand and the potential of offering yoga for well-being, Mona founded The Yoga Connection, a 501c3 nonprofit which provides empowerment and community to immigrant and refugee women through a group yoga therapy class. In addition to workshops and retreats, Mona offers an evidence-based course, Trauma-Sensitive Training for Mind-Body Professionals, with example modules focused on the immigrant population. Mona was the recipient of the 2020 International Association for Yoga Therapists Seva Award. To learn more about Mona, her services, teachings, and retreats, visit www.lifefityoga.com.